T·A·K·E C·O·N·T·R·O·L S·E·R·I·E·S

STROKE!
a self-help manual for relatives and carers
Dr R. M. Youngson

**Books supplying expert information and practical
guidance to help YOU take control**

Titles published so far include

ALCOHOLISM
an insight into the addictive mind
Dr Clive Graymore

·

FERTILITY
a comprehensive guide to natural family planning
Dr Elizabeth Clubb and Jane Knight

·

SCHIZOPHRENIA
a fresh approach
Gwen Howe

·

DRUG ABUSE
the truth about today's drug scene
Tony Blaze-Gosden

·

HEALTH DEFENCE
Dr Caroline Shreeve

STROKE!

a self-help manual
for stroke sufferers
and their relatives

Dr R. M. Youngson

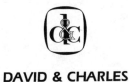

DAVID & CHARLES
Newton Abbot   London

British Library Cataloguing in Publication Data

Youngson, R. M.
  Stroke! a self help manual for stroke
  sufferers and their relatives. – (Take
  control)
  1. Cerebrovascular disease – Patients
  – Rehabilitation
  I. Title   II. Series
  362.1'9681   RC388.5

  ISBN 0-7153-8945-9

Typeset by Typesetters (Birmingham) Ltd,
Smethwick, West Midlands
Printed in Great Britain
by A. Wheaton & Co Ltd   Hennock Road   Exeter
for David & Charles Publishers plc
Brunel House   Newton Abbot   Devon

Distributed in the United States
by Sterling Publishing Co, Inc,
2 Park Avenue, New York, NY 10016

Contents

Preface

Suffering, and surviving, a stroke is one of the most frightening and distressing things that can happen to anyone. Often without any warning, normal life is torn apart by the sudden loss of basic bodily or mental function – movement, speech, understanding, sensation or vision. In the most severe strokes the victim is mercifully spared this distress and knows little of what has happened. Consciousness and awareness are deeply impaired and only the onlooker is distressed. But to the sufferer with less severe brain damage, the physical effects are likely to have horrifying implications for his future life. He may see his career shattered, his earning power drastically cut, his ambition frustrated, or his hopes for an active and rewarding retirement destroyed. There is a dreadful sense of helplessness, and of loss of control over his own destiny, and the effect on morale is devastating. For the relatives, too, and especially for the person left mainly in charge, there is bewilderment and uncertainty. The thing that has happened is often beyond comprehension, and the possibility of actually being able to do anything useful seems remote. Again, there is a frightening sense of helplessness.

But in neither case is this feeling wholly justified. Knowledge and understanding can, to a surprising extent, dispel fear. And, with good advice and sound information much may be salvaged from what may seem to be the wreckage of a life. This book is one of a series called 'Take Control'. In this case the title has an extra dimension of meaning, for it applies both to the stroke victim and to those who have to look after him. Much of the book is addressed directly to the carer – often the wife or husband of the person who has had the stroke – but, for those sufferers from stroke illness able to read and understand it, there is also a great deal in it. The book looks at every important aspect of the condition, which is very important if the fullest possible degree of recovery is to be achieved. For in stroke illness, perhaps more than in any other serious condition, the degree of recovery depends to a remarkable extent on the motivation, determination and hope of the sufferer.

The central purpose of this book is to provide these essential ingredients.

Dr R M Youngson

1 Warnings

WHO GETS STROKE, AND WHY?_____

If stroke is to be understood, some background explanations are necessary and this chapter, and the next, will provide them. But although intended as a general introduction to the subject, this information could be of the greatest importance to the reader – especially if middle-aged and a close relative of someone who has had a stroke. These preliminary chapters deal with the warning signs so that suitable precautions can be taken to avoid the same fate. Even if the reader has already had a stroke it is essential that these things should be known, for strokes can, and do, recur and every recurrence can add to the disability.

This is not a medical textbook and no medical knowledge is needed to understand it. Some medical terms are used, but all of these are explained. The story of what happened to two people who experienced these warnings will help to make everything plain.

Joe Grouse and his transient ischaemia

Joe was a forty-seven year old systems analyst working for a major software house specialising in producing computer systems for hospital patient administration. He was good at his job, which involved making a detailed analysis of the requirements of hospitals using large computers, and progressively up-dating the systems. He spent a lot of time talking to hospital staff and studying their requirements.

One day when, by pure coincidence, he happened to be talking to a Consultant Physician about extending the disease indexing facility, he became aware that his thoughts had become confused and that he had lost the thread of what he was saying. At the same time a most extraordinary thing happened to his vision – the right half of everything he looked at seemed to have disappeared. Then he noticed that his right arm seemed to have lost almost all its power. Embarrassed and alarmed, and anxious to give himself time to think, he managed to fumble a cigarette out of its packet, using his left hand, lit it and took a deep drag.

The consultant was looking at him curiously. 'Are you all right?' he asked.

'Half which . . . sorry machine code . . .' said Joe. He felt for a chair and sat down suddenly. With a trembling hand, he put the cigarette to his mouth and pulled the smoke down into his lungs. For a moment he wasn't sure whether he was going mad or was about to die. Then he noticed that his vision to the right was beginning to come back again and with a sense of unutterable relief he realised that his thoughts were becoming ordered once more. Almost afraid to try, he began to speak.

I'm . . . sorry,' he said slowly, 'I don't know what came over me.' He held up his right hand and flexed his fingers. Then he covered one eye at a time and looked around.

The consultant held out both his hands. 'Grab my fingers,' he said, 'Grip as hard as you can.'

Joe looked surprised but did as he was asked.

'Checking your muscle power,' explained the consultant, 'Seeing if the strength is the same in both hands.'

'And is it?'

'Just about. Maybe a little weaker on the right.'

He unhooked the stethoscope from his neck, put the ear-pieces in his ears, and leaned forward and pressed the bell of the instrument firmly to the right side of Joe's neck.

'What . . .?'

The consultant listened to the left side of Joe's neck. After a moment he sat back. 'How are you feeling, now?' he asked.

'Scared . . . but better. How did you know my arm . . .?'

'Your speech was confused. That's called aphasia. And I noticed that you were checking the vision in both eyes –'

'So? What does that mean?' Joe looked around but there were no ash trays.

'You've had a transient ischaemic attack – a TIA – and you're going to need a full work-up.'

'Is it serious – a TIA?'

'Not in itself. But it's a warning that you ignore at your peril.'

'Of what?'

'Of a stroke.'

'My God! D'you mean that?' Joe opened his packet with trembling fingers and took out another cigarette.

'Certainly. Actually, you're quite lucky. Lots of people have a stroke without anything they can recognise as a warning at all. There nearly always *is* warning, but not usually as dramatic as that. Do you have to smoke that cigarette?'

Joe put the cigarette back in the packet. 'What's 'ischaemic'?'

'Insufficiency of blood to any part of the body. In this case, a part of the brain.'

'Oh!'

'As you know, body tissues simply must have oxygen and sugar if they are to work properly. The main function of the blood circulation is to transport these two vital supplies to all parts. The sugar is the fuel and the oxygen is needed to oxidise it so that energy can be released. The blood picks up oxygen from the lungs and sugar from the gut or liver and carries them to the tissues. The brain is acutely sensitive to oxygen lack and any reduction in the blood supply is a serious matter –'

'Well, how can that happen?'

'Oh, in several ways and we'll be checking, in your case, to find out the actual cause – whether narrowing of blood vessels, thrombosis, embolus or whatever.'

'Hang on! Can you explain?' Joe asked.

The consultant glanced at his watch. 'Normally I wouldn't have time,' he said, 'but you've caught me on my admin. afternoon.'

'Well, thanks.'

'OK,' said the physician. 'Your brain is your most important organ and it's the best protected. In a way the whole of the rest of the body can be considered as simply a means of supporting the brain and carrying out its decisions. Your heart, on the other hand, is a powerful mechanical pump, with valves, to keep the blood going round, and, most importantly of all, to maintain the supply of blood to your brain. Cut off the supply of blood to the brain for more than about three minutes, at normal temperatures, and irreparable brain damage occurs. Cut off the supply for more than eight minutes and death is inevitable.'

'Yes, I knew about that. But why?'

'Nerve tissue has such a high energy requirement that it actually dies if oxygen isn't constantly available.'

'So nerve tissue is functioning all the time?'

'Yes, and if it were to stop, you would, too – very quickly. So – to proceed. Out of the top of the heart comes a very large artery called the aorta, which arches over in a sharp curve and runs down alongside the spine, giving off branches to all parts. The first two branches, coming off immediately above the heart are the coronary arteries which spread over the heart muscle like a crown – 'coronary' means a crown – and supply the muscle itself with essential blood.'

'You're talking about the arteries that are affected in coronary thrombosis?'

'Yes. But it's the next group of arteries, branching off the aorta, that I'm really concerned with at the moment. These are four large trunks which come off on the top of the curve and run up the neck to supply the head. Two of these actually make their way up through a succession of holes in the side processes of the bones of the spine – the vertebrae – so they are called the vertebral arteries. The other two are larger and nearer the front and are called the carotids – the name comes from a Greek word meaning 'to stupefy'. If you squash these arteries against the spine, so as to cut off the blood flow, the victim becomes unconscious and dies.'

'These four arteries, the carotid arteries and the vertebrals, are absolutely essential to provide the large requirements of nutrition to the brain and if they are diseased you could be in trouble.

'Is there something wrong with my arteries?'

'It's likely you have the number one killer – atherosclerosis – and that this is affecting your carotids. They could be narrowed. That's why I listened with the stethoscope – to see if there was a whooshing noise as the blood went through a narrowed vessel –'

'And was there?'

'A bit, I'm afraid. But that's not conclusive. There are other causes.'

'What was that thing you think I have.'

'Atherosclerosis. It's a combination of arteriosclerosis – hardening of the arteries – and a condition called atheroma.'

'You'd better explain.'

'Atherosclerosis is by far the largest single cause of death in the world. In fact, atherosclerosis causes as many deaths as all the other causes put together. So it's important. The two main ways it causes death are by affecting the arteries supplying the heart – the coronary arteries – so as to cause coronary thrombosis, and the arteries supplying the brain – the carotids and vertebrals and their smaller branches. What atherosclerosis does is to lay down fatty material in the inner lining of the arteries so that they not only become narrowed but are also prone to clotting of the blood within them.'

'Is that a thrombosis?'

'Only if the clot blocks off the artery altogether. If the coronary arteries are much affected by atherosclerosis they are very prone to thrombosis. But sometimes the clot that forms is a bit loose and may be carried away in the bloodstream. This is called an embolus, and it is usually emboli that cause TIAs.'

'You mean emboli from clots in the carotid arteries?'

'Sometimes little bits of clotted blood can also come from the heart and this is quite common if there has been a small, perhaps unnoticed, coronary. This also tends to happen if there is disease of the heart valves, as occurs, for instance, in rheumatic fever. Sometimes quite young people get TIAs, or even strokes, if clots have formed on diseased heart valves.'

'Presumably a complete thrombosis of a carotid artery is pretty serious?'

'Actually, the system is very well designed and the branches of the carotids and vertebrals which supply the brain don't just peter out into smaller and smaller twigs. Instead, they join up together to form a circle of arteries surrounding the stem of the brain, so that branches coming from this circle receive blood from all four sources.'

'You mean, one carotid could be blocked and the brain could still get enough blood?'

'That's right – assuming that one carotid and the two vertebrals were healthy and capable of carrying a full blood-flow. Unfortunately, if a person has atherosclerosis, all the arteries are likely to be affected to a greater or lesser degree.'

'I see. So my carotids are pretty narrow?'

'I don't really know yet. We'll be doing an arteriogram to find out.'

'Is that some kind of X-ray?'

'Yes. It's a new way of showing up the state of the insides of arteries. It's a sort of scanner that compares two pictures taken before and after injecting an X-ray opaque dye into the blood-stream. One picture is turned into a negative to cancel all the information – like the images of the bones – that is identical in both pictures. So only the difference shows up and that is the dye in the blood. This, of course, fills the available internal space in the blood vessels and shows exactly what's going on. It's called a subtraction arteriogram and it will tell us whether your trouble is in the carotids.'

'Why doesn't blood clot in normal arteries? It clots as soon as it's spilt, doesn't it?'

'Yes. But then it comes in contact with various foreign materials including tissue fluid from the cut edges of the bleeding vessel and that starts a complex biochemical process ending in the formation of a clot. If you put blood carefully into a very clean, wax-coated tube it will not clot. Normally, the inner linings of the blood vessels are very smooth and the substances needed to start the clotting reaction are absent. But atheroma encourages clots to form. The same applies to injury, from any cause, to the vessel lining. For instance, when someone has had a small coronary thrombosis, the inner lining of the heart itself may be damaged to the point where blood starts to clot there. This is a very common source of emboli and about one case of stroke in five is caused by emboli from the inside of the heart following coronary thrombosis.'

'Are you saying that these people have a coronary *and* a stroke?'

'Yes. About ten per cent of strokes are caused that way.'

'Do some people have blood that clots more easily than others?'

'Yes. All sorts of things can alter the strength of the tendency of the blood to clot. The contraceptive pill, for one thing. A lot of strokes in young women have been attributed to that. There's no doubt that the pill does affect coagulation. Women on the pill also get vein thromboses. Pregnancy, too, is a dangerous time.'

'What else affects blood clotting?'

'Oh, major injury, surgical operations, cancer. Several other things.'

'And you think I've had a clot come away from somewhere and go up to my brain?'

'It may have been a clot, or it may have been some fatty material from a patch of atheroma – perhaps even a crystal of pure cholesterol. Whatever it was, it lodged in a smallish vessel in the left side of your brain, probably a branch of the middle cerebral artery –'

'Why the left side?'

'Two reasons. It affected your speech – and I see that you're right handed, so the left hemisphere is the dominant one. Also, the slight weakness was on the right, and the left side of the brain controls the right side of the body.'

'I see. So what happened to the clot – or embolus, or whatever? Has it gone away?'

'No. I'm afraid not.'

'Well, how is it that I recovered?'

'The area of brain supplied by the blocked artery is now being supplied by other, smaller arteries that have opened up to make up the supply. This is called establishment of a collateral circulation.'

'I don't like the sound of that,' said Joe, 'Presumably that part of the brain now has less reserve.'

'Yes. If you were unlucky enough to have another fairly large embolus in the same area, it might go badly with you. A transient ischaemic attack is one in which the loss of neurological function begins suddenly, persists for less than twenty-four hours – usually only a few minutes – and clears without leaving any obvious disability. But in about fifteen per cent of people who have had a TIA there is a demonstrable area of permanent brain damage – very small, of course.'

'How do you mean – demonstrable?'

'It can be seen on a CT scan as a patch of dead tissue.'

'Good God!'

'Lots of people have large numbers of TIAs with little or no apparent disability. It's entirely a matter of the size of the embolus. A large embolus will not produce a TIA. It will produce a stroke, with damage varying from minor to total.'

'What's worrying me is this,' said Joe, 'What's to stop this happening again? If my carotid arteries are both narrowed, presumably the vertebral arteries are also affected –'

'Possibly –'

'Isn't that dangerous?'

'Well, it's not to be recommended. Severe carotid narrowing is a very common cause of strokes, even without emboli. Indeed, the majority of strokes occur simply from not enough blood getting to the brain.'

'So what happens next?' asked Joe.

'You need a full workup and I think it would be best if you came in for a few days so that this can be done properly – and as quickly as possible.'

'Absolutely!'

'There are two things you can do to help yourself.'

'What's that? I'll do anything –'

'One is to stop smoking. Right now.'

Joe looked stricken. 'But I don't see how that can –'

'Listen,' said the consultant, 'and listen hard. Thousands of post-mortem examinations have shown that smokers have much more atherosclerosis than non-smokers – especially in the aorta and the carotids. Smoking increases the heart rate and raises the blood pressure – both factors which cause atherosclerosis. High blood pressure is one of the main risk factors for stroke. Smoking causes increased adhesiveness between certain cells in the blood necessary for clotting and definitely increases the tendency. The carbon monoxide you inhale with the smoke cuts down the ability of your blood to carry oxygen to a significant degree. So, if you are in a border-line situation smoking could tip the balance. You could, quite literally, smoke yourself to death. You want to hear any more?'

'No,' he said, weakly, 'I've got the message. What was the other thing I should do?'

'When we were talking about blood clotting, I was concerned with the factors that encourage it. There are some things one can do to *discourage* clotting, and probably the most useful is to take a very small dose of aspirin – I suggest you take one 'baby' aspirin every day.'

'And that will help?'

'Yes. Aspirin affects the platelet stickiness. It can even prevent any more TIAs.'

Joe Grouse's medical work-up

Joe was admitted to hospital the same day. His mind was whirling with the dire possibilities suggested by the consultant physician's bland account of the causes of stroke and he kept going through the list, wondering which would apply to him. Could he have had a small coronary and produced a blood clot inside his heart? He *had* been having occasional pain in the chest, but he had just put it down to indigestion or maybe the smoker's cough that he had had for years. Could he have some problem with his heart valves? That seemed unlikely but he would almost rather that that was the case then that he had severe narrowing of his carotid arteries. He didn't really want to think about his carotid arteries. The idea of being slowly strangled didn't appeal to him at all.

The consultant's senior registrar was more relaxed in manner than his boss and Joe felt more at ease with him. 'Is smoking really so dangerous?' he asked.

'God, yes! It's not so much the risk of lung cancer, although that's serious enough. I'd be more worried about respiratory and cardio-vascular effects –'

'Cardio-vascular?'

'Heart and blood vessels,' said the doctor, 'Coronary thrombosis and atherosclerosis. I used to smoke, but now I can't stand the thought of it. I hate even inhaling other people's smoke and I really resent having to do that in enclosed places.'

'I'm dying for a fag,' said Joe, 'Look at the way my hands are shaking.'

'A fag might be what you literally are dying for. And you wouldn't be the first. I've seen some horrible results from smoking. I tell you, I hate cigarettes!'

Joe changed the subject. 'What's on the agenda?' he asked, trying to sound cheerful.

'Well, we're especially interested in the condition of your arteries and we'll be checking your heart and blood pressure. You'll be having an electrocardiogram. Of course, we'll be doing a full blood check and that will include a check of the thickness of the blood as well as fasting cholesterol and triglyceride levels. And we'll check for diabetes. Probably most important of all, you'll be having angiography of the arteries supplying your brain –'

'The carotids and the vertebrals.'

'That's right. You've been lucky enough to have a TIA and early investigation, so the risks, for you, are not all that great . . .'

'Are you going to tell me just how much danger I'm in?' asked Joe quietly.

'Do you really want to know?'

'Yes, I do.'

'Well, the figures show that after the first TIA there is about one chance in twenty of a stroke occuring in the first year. I'm afraid that for most patients this risk continues – that is, about five per cent of them get a stroke each year.'

'Oh well,' said Joe, 'Now I know. What about the risk of death? I suppose that's much less?'

The doctor hesitated. 'Well no,' he said, 'It's about the same. Five per cent per year.'

'But that doesn't make sense,' said Joe, 'unless every stroke is fatal.'

'The explanation is that more people in this group die from coronary thrombosis than from stroke.'

'Really! Isn't that rather strange?'

'No. Atherosclerosis causes many more deaths from coronaries than from strokes. The coronary arteries are terribly susceptible to blockage from thrombosis and if a person has had TIAs he is likely to have generalised atherosclerosis.'

Joe rubbed his chest. 'I'm more likely to get a coronary than a stroke, is that right?'

'Yes. Especially if you go on smoking.'

THE SIGNIFICANCE OF HIGH BLOOD PRESSURE

The medical workup produced two findings of note – angiography showed that Joe's left carotid artery was almost occluded by a large atherosclerotic plug, and repeated measurements showed that his blood pressure was much higher than it should have been.

'I don't really understand about blood pressure' said Joe to the Registrar, 'Can you tell me why it's dangerous?'

'Sure. If you take a lot of people with pressures above normal, divide them into two equal groups and treat one group so as to bring the blood pressures down to normal, you will find, over the course of the next few years, that there are far fewer cases of stroke in the treated group than in the untreated. You will also find many fewer cases of coronary thrombosis.'

'Why is that?'

'High blood pressure and atherosclerosis are closely linked. This isn't really surprising. Obviously, elastic arteries can stretch and give a little so that the pressure is reduced. Sometimes the arteries are so rigid that with each heart beat the pressure rises very steeply indeed.'

'Does the pressure ever burst the arteries?' asked Joe.

'Sure. Sometimes, if the smaller arteries are very hardened one of them may be unable to resist the pressure and bursts. The haemorrhage that results may not matter very much in some parts of the body, but, inside the skull, and especially inside the brain, the effect may be devastating. Cerebral haemorrhage causes the most serious kinds of strokes and many patients who suffer cerebral haemorrhage die from the first episode. Fortunately, the majority of strokes are not caused in this way and, as I've said, by finding out that you have high blood pressure, and getting it treated, you can greatly reduce the risk of this happening. The worst combination of all is high blood pressure and smoking. This carries a particularly high risk of developing stroke and coronary thrombosis.'

'So you'll be treating my blood pressure, will you?' Joe asked, 'What causes high blood pressure, anyhow?'

'Oh, there are lots of factors. Heredity is one – I mean, if your parents had it you are more likely to get it. Excessive weight is another. Cigarette smoking. Kidney disease can cause it. Stress. An aggressive personality. Excess cholesterol in the blood. Possibly too much salt in the diet. Lack of exercise. The pill – lots of things. But the most important are smoking and the development of atherosclerosis. Diet and exercise are obviously important.'

Joe ran his hand over his pot belly.

About two weeks after entering hospital Joe was taken to theatre where a delicate operation was performed on his left carotid. The tests had shown that the other carotid and the two vertebrals were much less affected, so the surgeon felt that it would be safe to clamp off the affected artery and rely on the blood getting around the linking channels from the other vessels. This proved to be so. After the artery had been clamped above and below the position of the obstruction, it was carefully opened, by a longitudinal incision, and the atherosclerotic plaque shelled out. When this had been done, the artery was closed again with ultra-fine silk stitches and the clamps removed.

Joe never looked back. His recovery was uneventful, and angiography, done afterwards showed that the blood flow in the artery which had been operated upon was now entirely normal.

'You've come through a pretty major operation with flying colours,' said the vascular surgeon, 'Do you propose to continue with exactly the same lifestyle? Because, if you do, you'll be as bad as ever in a couple of years.'

'Do you think I'm crazy?' asked Joe. 'This is day one of my new life. No smoking. Low fat diet. Weight control. Plenty of exercise.'

The surgeon smiled. 'Well, we'll see,' he said, 'Maybe you've got more sense than all the others.'

MORE ABOUT TIAs

The more you know about transient ischaemic attacks the better. TIAs may occur only once or twice in a year, or may occur many times a day, but unless the cause is removed, they *are* likely to recur. A person having TIAs has a fifty per cent chance of having a full stroke within five years of the start of the symptom. This is a rather horrifying finding and indicates how important it is to recognise TIAs and seek early treatment.

Remember that a TIA is a brief disturbance of *any* of the many functions of the brain. So, a TIA may cause brief loss of half of the field of vision in both eyes (involvement of the visual part of the brain, at the back), dizziness or faintness, vertigo, confusion of thought, loss of speech or of the understanding of the meaning of words or of the names of objects, weakness or numbness of one side of the body or even temporary loss of consciousness. Vision can be disturbed in another way. Tiny emboli can get into an eye, by way of the blood supply, and can cause temporary loss of function of part of the retina. In this case, of course, only one eye will be affected. This is quite a common form of TIA – commoner than visual field loss.

This list is not complete, but covers the great majority of effects. *Any* transient symptom which could be attributed to disturbance of brain action should be considered as a TIA until proved otherwise by medical examination.

Some of these symptoms – especially faintness and vertigo and occasional forgetfulness – are caused much more commonly by innocent causes than by TIAs, and one must view the matter intelligently. Remember also, that migraine often produces symptoms which are identical to those of a TIA. This is because migraine involves a spasm of the brain blood vessels, lasting for about twenty minutes, and this can cause all sorts of effects which are nearly always quite harmless. In fact, by providing a sort of 'trailer' of what may happen in a stroke, migraine can be a most educative, if sometimes alarming, experience.

TIAs become commoner with advancing age – about one person in five hundred over the age of sixty-five has them – and the younger the age at which they occur, the more serious the significance. TIAs occurring below the age of sixty are more likely to be followed by a serious stroke than those occurring in older people. Millions of people have had TIAs and have got away with it. But to ignore them is the height of foolishness. To be forewarned is to be forearmed.

Mrs Bliss was not so lucky

People with threatened stroke may present to specialists in various disciplines. Most are seen by GPs or by physicians, but referral to neurologists, neuro-surgeons and to eye specialists is common. This is how I came to meet Mrs Bliss. She was a delightful person, well-preserved, in her late fifties, lively and attractive and able to express herself clearly. She said she had only come because her GP had insisted.

I asked her to sit down and tell me what had been worrying her.

'I didn't believe, at first, that my headaches had anything to do with my eyes, but in the past two or three weeks my vision has been quite severely blurred and I'm beginning to wonder.

'Tell me about the headaches.' I said.

'They're quite different from ordinary headaches. For one thing I get them while I'm sleeping and they actually wake me up in the mornings.'

'Every morning?'

'Well, yes. Recently anyhow.'

'Where is the pain?'

'Everywhere. All over my head.'

'How would you describe it? What's it like?'

'It's a steady, pounding headache and my head feels as if it's going to burst.'

'Pounding? Like a pulse?'

'Yes. I wondered about that, so I felt my pulse and the headache beats at the same rate.'

'Are there any other symptoms?'

'Well, I've noticed that I get breathless much more easily than I used to and I often feel terribly giddy.'

'Are these new symptoms?'

'Oh yes. Only for the last month or so.'

'And you never had them before?'

'No, never.'

'Do you have to walk more slowly than you used to?'

'Yes,' she said, then smiled, 'But I just put that down to age.'

'Tell me about the blurring of vision.'

'Well, I naturally assumed that it was my glasses needing changing, but I was a bit upset, because I've never needed glasses for distance – only for reading.'

'And did you get new glasses?'

'Yes. But they didn't make a bit of difference. Very expensive they were, too.'

'Is the blurring all over your field of vision?'

'No. I can see all right straight ahead, but I don't seem to see nearly so well to the left side –'

'To the left side with each eye separately?'

'No. It's really my left eye that's affected. The right one seems quite normal.'

When I tested her vision I found that, on the left side it was only about one quarter of normal (6/18) and, on the right, about half normal (6/12). Then I had a look inside her eyes with an ophthalmoscope and, at once, the cause of her trouble was clear. The optic nerve heads – which are clearly visible at the back of the inside of the eyes – were swollen and surrounded by flame-shaped patches of free blood. Similar haemorrhages were scattered about on both her retinas and, in addition, I saw the ominous 'cotton-wool' spots, indicating that, already, parts of the retinas had been destroyed. The retinal blood vessels, emerging from the optic nerve, in each eye, were irregular and twisted. The whole picture was unmistakeable. Mrs Bliss was suffering from severe high blood pressure (hypertension) and was at considerable risk from stroke.

'Roll up your sleeve, please,' I said neutrally, reaching for the sphygmomanometer.

As I wrapped the cuff carefully round her upper arm, she said, 'I wondered if it might be blood pressure . . .'

Mrs Bliss's running pressure, between heart beats (diastolic pressure) was 116 millimeters of mercury, and with each beat of her heart the pressure (systolic pressure) shot up to an alarming 210.

'Yes,' I said, 'I'm afraid that's the cause of the trouble.'

'Is it bad?'

'Pretty bad. I'll want you in hospital right away.'

'To tell you the truth,' she said, 'I'm quite relieved. I've been terribly worried. I'm so glad something is being done.'

Regrettably, we didn't have time to do anything. While I was writing up her admission notes, Mrs Bliss suffered a massive stroke, with complete paralysis down the right side of her body and deep coma. She was taken at once to the intensive care ward, but the coma was rapidly deepening and, as she was being lifted on to the bed, she died.

When I heard the news, I thought, bitterly, 'Why didn't she come earlier? She could easily have been saved, if she had come sooner.' But Mrs Bliss was the sort of person who didn't like to trouble anyone, and, right to the end, she was very little trouble.

2 TIAs, Thrombosis and Haemorrhage

THE CAUSES OF TRANSIENT ISCHAEMIA

Joe was lucky. Some people, like Mrs Bliss, don't even have transient ischaemic attacks (TIAs) to warn them of a stroke. As suggested, there will almost always be some indication that the state of health leaves something to be desired, but many people ignore symptoms and just hope for the best. Some may even fail to notice quite severe symptoms and may be struck down with paralysis and other damage as the first indication that anything is wrong. Ideally, of course, we should all have regular medical check-ups including careful history-taking and full examination to bring out any such symptoms. Regular checks of the blood-pressure, heart, lungs, and laboratory tests of the blood and urine are all of immense value in protecting against catastrophe.

Fortunately, TIAs are common enough to provide us with some warning and it is very important to recognise them and appreciate their significance. TIAs are caused by temporary shut-down in the blood supply to part of the brain and this may be due to nothing more than a general narrowing of all the arteries, so that the supply is precarious and cannot meet additional demands. Obviously, some arteries will tend to be more narrowed than others, so certain parts of the brain will be at greater risk. But most TIAs are the result of small particles of material in the blood, which ought not to be there at all. These particles are called emboli (each one is an embolus) and the more known about them the better.

EMBOLI

Old Mrs Molyneux had known for ages that there was something wrong with her eyes. Most of the time she could see perfectly well and she was normally delighted with the quality of her colour TV. But every now and then the vision of one eye would fog over – usually for a few seconds at a time, but sometimes for several minutes – and during these periods she would be convinced that she was going blind. The attacks would occur once or twice a day for about ten days and would then go away altogether for two or three months only to come back again. Each time she decided to go to her doctor the attacks would stop and she would let it go, hoping that the trouble would not return.

But her eyes were not the only thing worrying Mrs Molyneux. There were the dizzy spells – often occurring when her eyes were worst affected – so severe that she had to hold on tight to her chair. Sometimes she had short periods of double vision and these worried her terribly. It was unfortunate that she did not consult her doctor, for Mrs Molyneux was very much at risk and there was a simple explanation of her symptoms. Like many people at risk of stroke, Mrs Molyneux was producing in her bloodstream showers of small free emboli and these were being carried up the carotid and vertebral arteries to her brain. She took no action, but continued to hope for the best and, in the end, suffered a major stroke.

Small emboli consist of different kinds of material and are not actual blood clots like larger emboli. Many of them – especially those that form in the heart – are made up of fibrin tangled up with tiny blood cells called platelets. Platelets and fibrin are essential for blood clotting and it is this combination which forms spontaneously on the inner surface of arteries, or on the inner lining of the heart chambers, if either have been damaged. In both cases, atherosclerosis is the commonest cause – either directly, in the case of the arteries, or indirectly by way of coronary thrombosis in the case of the heart lining.

Emboli can also be formed from the fatty plaques of atherosclerosis on the inside of the arteries. Quite often, these lumps of 'porridge' break up and release debris into the blood. Emboli of this type come only from the arteries, not from the heart. Although they are usually small and cause TIAs, they can be so large that they block major arteries and cause complete strokes or even death. It is quite common for pathologists to find large arteries in the brain clogged off with this material.

The third type of emboli consist of pure crystals of cholesterol. These are very tiny and are a common cause of TIAs. Happily, pure cholesterol emboli, unless present in enormous numbers, are unlikely to do serious harm. But, as we shall see, they do cause observable effects which are a clear warning and which must never be ignored.

TIAs AND VISION

One common indication of transient ischaemia is sudden disturbance of vision. This can occur in various ways, all of which we must be able to recognise. Knowing what this kind of symptom means can prompt us to seek early treatment and so can be life-saving. How does this symptom come about?

Like the brain, the eyes are very sensitive to lack of oxygen. On the inside of the back of each eyeball is a complex, transparent membrane called the retina. The lens system of the eye casts a sharp image on the retina which, in turn, converts this, much in the way a TV camera does, into nerve impulses which are carried back to the brain along the optic nerves. Any interference with the full supply of blood to the retina will at once cause a loss of vision and this will vary in extent depending on how much of the retina is affected. If, for instance, an embolus found its way from the carotid to the artery which supplies the eye and the surrounding structures, the embolus might land in one of the external eye muscles and no one would be any the wiser. But if, by chance, it went into the branch of the artery which supplies the retina, and caused a temporary blockage of this branch or of one of its smaller sub-branches on the retina, it would be apparent at once that something had happened to the vision of that eye. If the blockage happened in the main trunk of the retinal artery, the whole of the field of vision would be affected, but if only a small sub-branch was blocked, only part of the field would be lost.

The effect, which may last from a few seconds to a minute or so, is like a blind or veil being drawn down in front of the eye, blanking out the vision. There is no pain or discomfort, no watering, no headache. Simply a silent, partial or complete, loss of vision. Because the obstruction almost always breaks up and disperses, the blood is able to get through again and the function of the retina is restored. But if loss of function lasts for more than about an hour – and this applies to any part of the nervous system – some nerve tissue will inevitably have been destroyed.

Transient ischaemic attacks of this type usually indicate disease of the carotid artery. There is another type of TIA affecting vision which has a different significance. Although the optic nerves go from each eye to the brain they don't just run into the front of the brain but pass right through to the back, to the part where the blood supply comes mainly from the vertebral arteries. On their way back, the fibres in the optic nerves split so that each half of the brain becomes responsible for seeing only half of the complete field of vision. The left half of the brain 'sees' the right-hand half of the field of each eye, and the right half 'sees' the left half field. So, if the blood supply to one half of the back of the brain is interfered with, there will be partial loss of vision in *both* eyes. By covering each eye in turn, one would find that the outer half of the field of vision of one eye, and the inner half of the field of the other, were missing. If the field loss was of the left half of both eyes, then the right side of the brain would be affected. If the right half of the field of each eye was missing, this would indicate loss of function of the back of the left side of the brain.

Such an experience shows that the trouble is caused by a reduction in the blood supply of the *vertebral* arteries, rather than the carotid arteries. Remember that the vertebral arteries are so called because they run up actually within the bones of the neck part of the vertebral column. Some people can produce temporary loss of half the field of vision simply by turning their heads to one side. This is because, in so doing, vertebral arteries, already narrowed, are being compressed further so that the blood flow is reduced.

When the trouble is in the vertebral artery supply, visual loss is by far the most common symptom. This is because such a large proportion of the blood from the vertebral arteries is used to supply the visual part of the brain. Sometimes the interference with vertebral blood supply is so severe that *both* halves of the back of the brain are involved. In this case, of course, all vision will be temporarily affected. This will produce either a complete blackout of vision – a very alarming experience – or a veil over the vision, sometimes with islands of entirely normal vision within it.

When the carotid arteries are the main seat of the trouble, the commonest symptom is temporary weakness or loss of sensation of one side of the body. But visual disturbance – in this case from emboli affecting the retina – is still very common, perhaps second in frequency. The carotids supply mainly the middle and front part of each half of the brain, and it is these parts of the brain that are responsible for movement, sensation and speech.

CAN SMALL EMBOLI CAUSE PERMANENT EFFECTS?

Although emboli usually cause brief periods of functional loss this is not always so. Large emboli are always serious, sometimes fatal. The continuous production of small emboli is certain to have a cumulatively damaging effect and doctors recognise that this can cause a gradual deterioration of a patient's condition. With larger emboli, causing observable minor damage each time, a condition called 'stroke-in-evolution' can occur. This distressing process of progressive disability is, however, more commonly caused by severe narrowing of the major vessels supplying the brain.

Sometimes a small embolus remaining intact in an important position may cause permanent damage. In one instance a senior Army officer complained of an annoying blind patch in the lower and outer part of the field of vision of his right eye. External examination of his eyes showed nothing wrong, but inspection of his retina with an ophthalmoscope showed a tiny, bright yellow flake lodged at the branch of one of the tiny retinal arteries. Beyond this point, the retina was paler than usual and it was clear that the cholesterol crystal had cut off the blood supply to a part of the retina and destroyed its function. A check with a stethoscope, over the lower ends of his carotid arteries, just above the collar bones, revealed a loud, harsh blowing sound with each heart-beat. Needless to say, this patient went immediately for full medical investigation.

OTHER EARLY SYMPTOMS OF STROKE

There are more symptoms than might be imagined although *any* function of the brain may be affected if the blood supply is impaired. The most obvious effects are weakness of one half of the body, loss of sensation on one side, disturbances of speech and understanding, and visual upset. Also occurring less commonly, are vertigo, nausea and vomiting, headache, loss of hearing, loss of memory, gradual changes of both personality and intellect, difficulty in swallowing, drowsiness, loss of consciousness and, occasionally, epileptic fits.

Obviously any or all of these symptoms may arise from causes unconnected with the development of stroke and some of them occur quite commonly from much more innocent causes. But if these symptoms occur in association with TIAs it is probable that they are being caused by inadequate blood supply to the brain and it would be very foolish not to seek urgent medical attention.

DROP ATTACKS

Episodes in which a perfectly conscious person – usually elderly – suddenly falls to the ground for no apparent reason are known as drop attacks. The cause is uncertain and if they occur in isolation, without any other indication of threatened stroke, they are probably of no great consequence. But a person showing the signs of insufficiency in the vertebral artery supply – loss of visual half fields, vertigo, double vision, etc – will quite often also suffer drop attacks. In that case, these are almost certainly due to inadequate blood supply to the brain and should be taken as an additional warning. Drop attacks are mentioned here because many people with visual symptoms and vertigo do not suspect that they might be due to shortage of blood to the brain.

MIGRAINE AND STROKE

Some of the effects of migraine can be very alarming, especially when they happen for the first time, as they can quite closely mimic the symptoms of stroke. Although migraine is almost always harmless, it temporarily affects the brain in a very similar way in that some of the branches of the carotid or vertebral arteries undergo a temporary constriction so that the blood flow through them is markedly reduced.

Following the narrowing stage, the blood vessels become enlarged and this causes stretching of the walls of the vessels – a severely painful process. This, possibly together with muscle spasm, causes the headache. But it is the initial constriction which is important here. Many migraine sufferers can describe accurately what it is like to lose one half of the visual field, to suffer weakness down one side of the body, or to lose sensation in the hands or part of the face – particularly around the mouth.

Fortunately, the very great majority of people with migraine can be assured that these symptoms will only last for about twenty minutes. This is because the arterial spasm operates in a 'fail-safe' manner, cutting off blood to the muscles in the walls of the arteries so that eventually these muscles – which are responsible for the spasm – have to relax. Although it is very rare, permanence of these effects does sometimes occur. Certainly women taking the contraceptive pill who also suffer from migraine are probably at considerably more risk of this happening than others. This risk is further increased if the migraine is treated with the commonly used drug ergotamine. This drug, which acts strongly on the muscles in the blood vessel walls, helps to reduce the migraine by causing spasm of the vessels and this could, in certain circumstances, be dangerous.

The combination of ergotamine and the pill operated in the case of a highly athletic young woman – a champion basketball player – who suffered a migraine during a game and had to stop because of the loss of visual field. Unfortunately, this loss did not clear up as expected but became permanent. She was admitted to hospital and a CT scan (computer assisted tomography) showed that a large area of one half of the back part of her brain had been deprived of its blood supply long enough for permanent changes to occur. The affected part showed up as a lighter patch, indicating that the brain tissue was dead.

It should be emphasised that this is very rare and that of the millions of migraine sufferers in the world, only a very small number ever suffer permanent tissue damage. But if three separate causes of shut-down in the blood supply – migraine, increased blood clotting tendency from oral contraceptives and sustained spasm of the vessel wall muscles from ergot – are operating, the risk is increased.

CEREBRAL HAEMORRHAGE_____

At one time actual bleeding within the skull (cerebral haemorrhage) was considered the main cause of stroke. However, only about fifteen per cent of all strokes are caused in this way. Bleeding may occur within the substance of the brain or from one of the arteries on the outer surface. There are two main causes. The first – high blood pressure with atherosclerosis – we are already familiar with. But the second, although quite common, is rather surprising and not very well known outside medical circles. It is illustrated by the harrowing story of Jennifer Page.

Jennifer's berry-like swelling (berry aneurysm)
Jennifer was fortunate in her doctor, for although he had not at first suspected anything very serious and, indeed, had written me a letter asking for a routine appointment, he had second thoughts about the case that evening and telephoned me.

'Sorry to be a nuisance, and call you at home,' he said, 'but I'm not too happy about a young woman I saw today.'

'What's the story?'

'Lovely young girl. Twenty-seven, a secretary. Previously very healthy. Sudden onset of very severe headache three days ago. Says she's hardly ever had headache before.'

'Location?'

'Started at the front, then moved to the back. Really violent.'

'Neck stiffness?'

'Yes, slight. But what's really worrying me is that she's developed a bit of double vision.'

'Any physical signs?'

'Well, I'm not sure. It's hard to be certain, but I rather think her left pupil is larger than the right. And I had an impression that the left upper lid was drooping a little.'

'Listen,' I said, 'We have an emergency on our hands. You must get that girl into hospital right away. Tonight.'

'What do you think it is?' he asked.

'Aneurysm on the Circle of Willis – until proved otherwise.'

'Oh God! Of course! Will you be there?'

'I'll be there.'

When Jennifer came in, her condition had already deteriorated. She was clearly distressed and in severe pain, her head held far back and her left eye closed. Normally, a detailed history is taken but, in this case, the features so obviously indicated serious disease of the nervous system that it was barely necessary. She sat down and, with one finger, I gently pulled up the drooping upper. The pupil was widely dilated and one could see only a thin rim of iris.

'I know you're feeling terrible, but it's essential to examine you.' I said. 'Could you just keep your head still and follow my finger with your eyes?'

As she did this, I watched her eyes carefully. When she looked to the left, her eyes moved normally, but when she tried to look to her right, her left eye did not move past the mid position. She was able to look down a little, but the upward movement was very limited.

'I get terrible double vision when I look right,' she gasped, 'Better to let the lid droop. Can't you do something for my headache?'

It was obvious that she had a paralysis of the left oculomotor nerve – responsible for inward and upward the movement of the eye and upward movement of the upper lid. The dilated pupil was also a sign of paralysis of this nerve. It was equally obvious that this was an urgent job for a neuro-surgeon.

Jennifer's neck rigidity increased rapidly and her head was soon forced backwards so that her chin pointed up. A sample of her cerebrospinal fluid, taken by lumbar puncture between two of the bones low down in her spine, was coloured pink and a rapid analysis in the laboratory confirmed that there had indeed been bleeding under one of the layers of membrane – the arachnoid layer – that surround the brain.

The neuro-surgeon took one look at her and said, 'Better get on with angiography. We're in trouble.'

Angiography used to involve passing a fine tube up the arm artery into the main arterial trunk of the body – the aorta – and injecting dye, opaque to X-rays, so that it passed up the four main arteries supplying the head. X-ray pictures then showed the exact shape of the columns of blood within the arteries. This method is still used widely but is being rapidly superceded by safer and better methods using computer imaging.

The neuro-surgeon snapped the X-ray film on to the illuminated viewing box, pointed to a large, round white blob, sticking out from one of the arteries, and said, 'There's your aneurysm.'

My colleague was pointing out that Jennifer had a berry-like swelling on one of the arteries of the important circle of vessels underneath the brain, formed by the junction of the terminations of the two carotid and the two vertebral arteries. This swelling – an aneurysm – was the result of a basic weakness in the elastic tissue in the wall of the vessel so that gradually, under the influence of blood pressure, a sac-like swelling had formed on the artery.

Aneurysms do arise from sites of pre-existing weakness, but are much commoner with high blood pressure. Trouble from them can occur at any age, but is commonest after fifty. Women are affected rather more than men. 'Apoplexy' – the dramatic episode in which, in a state of intense emotion such as rage or sexual excitement, a person is suddenly struck down unconscious, is usually due to the rupturing of an aneurysm which has been gradually enlarging and thinning on one of the brain arteries. Many of us quite unwittingly, have such aneurysms but they do not all cause trouble.

A massive bleed from an aneurysm is likely to be fatal, as, under high arterial pressure, blood may be forced into the soft substance of the brain, causing massive destruction of vital nervous tissue. If the person survives, there is likely to be severe disability and the form this takes will depend on the part of the brain damaged and the extent of the destruction. Because the skull is unyielding, the release of blood causes a sharp rise in pressure within the cranium leading to a general compression of the brain which may be forced downwards so that the brain-stem, with its vital centres, is squashed into the large opening in the base of the skull. Compression of these centres – which are responsible for respiration and heart-beat – is a common cause of death.

The danger facing Jennifer was obvious. Her neck stiffness and head retraction were caused by irritation to the brain linings (meninges) by the leaking blood, and this was getting rapidly worse. The main danger was that there might be a sudden tearing of the wall of the aneurysm. Soon after the angiography Jennifer went into coma and the urgency became greater. Drugs were given to lower her blood pressure and she was also given an injection of a drug called aminocaproic acid which was reputed to encourage the laying down of fibrin in the aneurysm and so reduce the tendency to bleeding.

The neuro-surgeon did not have much expectation of success from this measure, and after an hour in which her condition continued to deteriorate, he said, 'I'm afraid the only thing to do, at this stage, is to tie off her left carotid.'

'Risky, isn't it?' I said.

'Of course it's risky, but not so risky as leaving her. She's young. She'll have a good collateral circulation.'

At operation, the left carotid artery was exposed in Jennifer's neck and followed up to where the internal branch came off. A sterile tape was put round this branch and it was brought gently into clearer view. Then a clamp was applied and very carefully and slowly tightened so as to cut off the left internal carotid supply as gradually as possible.

'What are her chances?' I asked him afterwards.

'Tell you in the morning.' he said.

Jennifer's aneurysm stopped bleeding and she soon recovered consciousness and showed little sign of brain disfunction. There was a slight, temporary weakness of the right side of her body and a short period in which her speech was confused, but these soon passed and three weeks after the tying off of the carotid it was considered safe to perform the more difficult operation of tying off the aneurysm itself so as to make it safe and relieve the pressure on the nerve to the eye muscles. This was accomplished and, although she did not recover full mobility of the eye, it was possible, later, to improve things further by squint surgery.

I asked the neuro-surgeon about the mortality rate of bleeding aneurysms.

'Bloody awful.' he said, 'About half of them die. So we were quite lucky with Jennifer.'

INTERNAL BRAIN HAEMORRHAGE

Bleeding inside the substance of the brain is a common cause of stroke and is always associated with atherosclerosis and high blood pressure. Although the artery concerned is nearly always quite small, the result of the free squirting of blood within the brain is usually catastrophic. Stokes caused in this way usually occur when the person is awake. There is usually severe head pain and terrible dizziness and the full effects are apparent often within a few minutes – at the most, within an hour or so.

Many patients lose consciousness and rapidly develop severe weakness or paralysis of the side of the body opposite the side of the bleed. But this does not necessarily occur. There is often vomiting and neck stiffness and, quite commonly, fits. Usually the eyes remain turned to the side away from the paralysis or there may be inability to turn the eyes in a particular direction, and one pupil, or both, may be widely dilated. But bleeding may occur into half a dozen different sites within the brain and these will produce different effects, depending on the part damaged.

Cerebral haemorrhage has a death rate of from fifty to seventy five per cent. Many patients, like the unfortunate Mrs Bliss, die on the day of the bleed and the majority die within a month. Most of those who are in coma from the beginning never recover consciousness. But if a person does survive there is a very reasonable possibility of recovery. Much of the functional loss in the early stages is due, not to destruction of brain tissue, but to swelling and compression causing temporary loss of nerve conduction which is restored once the free blood has reabsorbed and the pressure on the nerve tracts is released. So the extent of the disability is always greatest at the beginning and some restoration of function usually occurs in those who survive.

It is encouraging that with proper treatment of the blood pressure, further bleeding can almost always be avoided. This is because of the small size of the vessels concerned in internal brain bleeding and the fact that such vessels can seal themselves off by the clotting of blood at the site of rupture.

HIGH BLOOD PRESSURE

Apart from aneurysm, the principle cause of cerebral haemorrhage is high blood pressure (hypertension) and this is a major risk factor for stroke. Mrs Bliss had very obvious hypertension, causing quite severe symptoms, and if she had been less considerate of other people, she might have had something done about it in time. Most people with hypertension do not have symptoms, but the condition may still be severe enough to increase the risk substantially. About forty per cent of people with a moderate or severe rise in blood pressure may, if not treated, expect to die within five years. And many of these die of stroke.

The moral is clear. Life style should be adjusted to avoid hypertension, if at all possible. Regular blood pressure checks should be carried out and, if necessary, hypertension treated. But prevention is always better than cure, so how can we avoid this dangerous condition?

The first point concerns body weight. Obesity is so commonly associated with hypertension as to leave no doubt that it is to be avoided at all costs. Obese people *always* eat unwisely and excessively and their diet invariably contains a large proportion of saturated fats – mainly animal fats – which, are also definite factors in atherosclerosis. Blaming obesity on 'glands' or finding other explanations, avoids facing up to the fact that one eats too much. Many people have the misfortune to be brought up with an overeating tendency and, for these, the battle is hard and never-ending and the adjustments very difficult. Such people may deserve sympathy but this does not modify the uncompromising necessity to cut down on food intake of all kinds, especially fats. Dairy products, except in strict moderation, are dangerous to all of us and deadly to the obese.

The second controllable risk factor for hypertension is smoking. The evidence is not mere medical prejudice or vague statistics. It is hard, unequivocal proof obtained in the consulting room and on the post-mortem table. It is the evidence of rigid, unyielding arteries in smokers and elastic arteries in non-smokers. It is also evident in the death rates and causes of death in smokers compared with non-smokers. The

s-c

evidence is incontrovertible. Smoking is one of the major causes of ill-health and human misery and if this book achieves nothing more than stopping a few people from indulging in such a harmful habit, it will not have been written in vain.

3 The Effects of Stroke

The effects of stroke may vary widely – from a minor, and barely discernible, disability to the most devastating loss of function leading to early death. The severity depends on two factors – how much of the brain substance is damaged and which parts are involved. There are considerable 'silent' areas at the front of the brain which are not essential to life and whose function is not completely understood. Extensive damage in these areas may have little apparent effect, whereas quite minor damage in more vital areas will be very serious. Unfortunately, although the frontal, 'silent' areas of the brain are often involved in stroke, it is seldom that these alone are affected. Most of the obvious functions of the brain – voluntary movement, sensation, sight, smell, speech and hearing – have their central computing mechanisms on the outer layer of one or both of the large upper hemispheres. This outer layer is called the cerebral 'cortex' and the functions of the various areas of the cortex have been accurately mapped out by observing people with known areas of damage or disease.

Immediately behind the frontal parts of the brain are the outer layers which are responsible for voluntary movement (motor areas) and sensation (sensory areas). The nerve connections descending from these areas are amongst the most commonly affected in stroke.

HEMIPLEGIA

'Hemiplegia' means 'half paralysis' and this is the most obvious and best known of all the effects of stroke. The motor areas of the cortex are about half-way back along the surface and from these areas massive bundles of nerve fibres pass downwards through the substance of the brain, into the swollen brain stem and down the spinal cord, carrying messages to all the muscles of the body. But in the brain stem and the upper part of the spinal cord, all the great motor nerve trunks originating in the right half of the brain cross over to the left side of the spinal cord, and those on the left

...de cross over to the right side. As a result of this, if damage is caused to that part of the right half of the brain, concerned with voluntary movement, the paralysis will affect the left half of the body. If the left half of the brain is damaged, the paralysis will be on the right side.

These nerve fibres converge to form inverted pyramids as they descend and cross. This is called the 'pyramidal' system and is concerned with voluntary, skilled movement particularly of the fingers and hands. The other section of the motor system, although capable of bringing about some voluntary movement, is concerned primarily with the many unconscious and automatic movements like breathing, the heart beat, the automatic parts of eating and such functions as sex and sleeping. This 'extra-pyramidal' system starts in the same motor area of the brain as the pyramidal system, but the nerve fibres do not run directly down to the brain stem and cord. Instead, they make various detours to other parts of the brain – parts concerned with coordination and control – before running down into the spinal cord. These detours carry the extra-pyramidal fibres around that part of the brain most vulnerable to cerebral haemorrhage or inadequacy of blood supply. The extra-pyramidal connections are also more spread out than the direct, closely-packed pyramidal fibres. As a result, and fortunately, the extra-pyramidal system is much less likely to be knocked out than the pyramidal system.

This is of tremendous importance to the stroke victim who suffers a cerebral haemorrhage in the area through which the pyramidal tracts run and loses lost nearly all pyramidal function on one side. For, if the extra-pyramidal system is intact, there is the possibility of this system taking over, to some extent, the function of the pyramidal tracts. But it will not be able to do so unless the person concerned has proper treatment from the very beginning.

Since each half of the brain has its own pair of large arteries to supply it – the carotids and vertebrals – it would be quite a coincidence if *both* sides were damaged simultaneously, so it is very unusual for paralysis, or loss of sensation or visual loss, to affect the two sides equally. Let's look more closely at hemiplegia.

Obviously, the damage to nerve fibres carrying movement messages may vary in extent, so that the loss of power in the muscles to which they are connected may range from slight weakness to total paralysis. This variation will depend on the number of nerve fibres affected by the ischaemia or haemorrhage. In cerebral haemorrhage, the destruction will often be widespread, but in every case, the severity of the paralysis or weakness will be greatest at the onset and will, almost always, tend to get less with time. This is because although some of the fibres are permanently destroyed, many of them are able to resume their function once the swelling caused by the lack of oxygen has settled. But this is not the whole basis of recovery. It is now believed that closely adjacent nerve fibres, not previously used for the function now damaged, can partially take over. This is an important observation with a bearing on the degree of recovery possible and it also highlights the importance of correct training during the recovery period.

Loss of muscle power is not the whole story in hemiplegia. There is also usually loss of *sensation*, and this contributes to the disability. In addition, the paralysis of voluntary movement is often associated, paradoxically, with a strong tendency for the affected muscles to go into a tight involuntary contraction when stretched. This is known as 'spasm' or 'spastic paralysis' and it is due to the nerves from the muscles to the spinal cord, and from the cord to the muscle, being intact. Normally, the messages from the brain over-ride these local 'reflex arcs' but when higher control is lost, the local reflexes can take over and can operate powerfully. The result is that any local stimulus to the muscles – such as squeezing or stretching – will cause a strong reflex contraction via the spinal cord so that the arm, or leg, cannot relax or even be moved passively by someone else without difficulty.

It is essential that this spasm should not lead to permanent distortion. Without treatment, this may happen over the course of a year or more, and will lead to irremediable deformity. Treatment to prevent this is vital and should be started at the earliest possible moment. This is discussed in the next chapter. The following case illustrates what may happen if treatment of hemiplegia is neglected.

What happened to Mrs Gowers

Mrs Gowers was an unlucky woman. She had always had a bitter aversion to dependency and lived alone in a cold and gloomy detached house in Hampstead. She had an income several times her needs and hardly spent anything. Her one remaining relative was waiting with ill-concealed impatience for her money. Mrs Gowers had no illusions about her nephew's attitude and did not encourage his visits. But she believed that blood was thicker than water and had let him know that he was her heir.

One day the nephew let himself in and found that his aunt was still in bed. He called to her and she indicated that he should come into her bedroom. She was lying in a large bed, tightly clutching a bottle of smelling-salts in her right hand and glaring at him. Her left arm was lying limp.

'Well, well, auntie!' he said, cheerfully, 'What's up? Not like you to stay abed at this time. Anything I can do?'

'I'm perfectly all right.' she said, snappily, 'Just gone a bit weak in my left arm. I'll have to have a day or two in bed, that's all.' He noticed that her face seemed a bit crooked and that, when she spoke, her lips puffed out occasionally, so that the 'p's and 'b's were breathy.

'Look here, auntie. Are you sure you're O.K.? You don't seem quite right to me. Perhaps I should get a doctor . . .'

'I forbid it! I just want you to ask Mrs Poole if she could look in every day instead of twice a week. I need a few things . . . shopping . . . a bit of help. Tell her she'll get something extra for her trouble. You'll telephone her, won't you?'

'If that's what the old trout wants,' he thought, 'no skin off my nose.'

The result was that Mrs Gowers remained in bed, being ministered to by her daily woman, for nearly a year. At length, even Mrs Gowers' indomitable character could not prevail against her helper's growing anxiety and, finally a doctor was called.

Dr Martin was horrified at what he found. After a glance at the bed, he opened the window to dispel the smell of the bedsores he knew he would find. Mrs Gowers had a complete paralysis of her left side (left hemiplegia) and because she had had no proper positioning or passive movement of any of the joints on her left side for so many months, the spasm which had followed the paralysis had produced terrible contractures of the affected muscles. Her head was twisted to the left side and her left shoulder and arm were drooping. Her left elbow was permanently bent so that the forearm was turned inwards and her wrist and fingers bent into a claw-like shape. The doctor found it impossible to straighten her arm or raise her shoulder.

Her left leg was turned permanently outwards at the hip. Her foot was dropped so that it was almost in a straight line with her leg, but turned inwards. Her whole body was twisted and leaning to the left and, for months, she had had to be supported by a pile of pillows to prevent her from falling to the left side. After her initial resentment, she accepted the doctor's attention and admitted, reluctantly, that she had suffered agonies from pressure on her buttocks and hip bones until the bedsores had become so large as to destroy the sensation altogether.

'Who has been attending to you? Isn't there a nurse? Haven't you been registered with a GP?

'The truth is, doctor, that I've always prided myself on seeing to myself. I can't bear to be dependent on anyone else. I'm afraid I've become a stubborn old woman.'

The doctor shook his head, but said nothing.

When she had been moved to hospital for proper care and investigation it was found that the stroke had involved the pyramidal tracts only and that her extra-pyramidal motor system was intact. The doctors decided that it was better not to tell her that, had she had normal management following the stroke, all the permanent bodily deformity could almost certainly have been avoided and she would probably have been able to walk again. As it was, she would remain gravely disabled.

SENSORY LOSS

The loss of sensation commonly accompanying hemiplegia is much more serious than just an absence of feeling in the skin. The person concerned may not know, without looking, where a hand, foot, arm or leg is positioned in space and there may be an almost complete unawareness of one half of the body – even, surprisingly enough, a kind of denial of ownership of the affected limbs. There may be a serious alteration in body image and of its position in relation to other objects and a total inability to identify simple objects, such as a door key, by feeling them. Such sensory loss can cause serious disability and can make certain occupations impossible. It may also greatly increase the difficulties of those trying to promote the patient's recovery.

APHASIA

Loss of the ability to move one side of the body is the most obvious effect of stroke, but it is not necessarily the most serious or distressing. When stroke affects the right side of the body, damage has been done to the left half of the brain and it is almost always there that the centres for communication – speech, writing, reading, comprehension – are situated. 'Aphasia' is disorder of language ability and this may include, to a varying degree, the ability to understand or express spoken or written language. The ability to spell, do simple calculations or to tell the time may also be affected. The terms 'dysphasia' and 'aphasia' are often used interchangeably. Don't worry about the difference. They really mean the same thing.

It is important to distinguish between the upset of communication caused by a blocking of the input of information from that caused by the individual's inability to express information. Unfortunately, some strokes are followed by a defect of both comprehension and expression. After a stroke, some people are completely unable to speak, while others can speak fluently, although not always sensibly. The difference is entirely a matter of which part of the half-brain is affected. Careful studies have shown that if the damage is towards the front of the left half of the brain, there will be a problem in expressing information and possibly inability to speak at all. If the damage is towards the back, there will be no disturbance of the ability to speak, but, unfortunately, what is said may not convey the desired information.

Speech defect may be caused by intellectual disturbance or may be a purely mechanical difficulty in which the muscles of the tongue, lips and palate are affected so that normal speech is impossible. Eating may also be affected.

READING DIFFICULTIES

After a stroke, difficulty in reading (alexia) is quite common and may be due to actual brain damage or to other factors, such as visual disturbance (see below) or loss of the power of concentration.

True alexia results from the inability to make sense of consecutive letters or words. However, if letters or words are written vertically rather than horizontally, they can usually be more easily read. This observation has led to a method of reading training, using vertical orientation of words, which, if started early, can achieve good results.

Alexia and the associated 'agraphia' (difficulty in writing) may be present to varying degrees. Difficulty of this kind frequently also involves problems with numbers and, tragically, in the case of musicians, a loss of the ability to comprehend musical notation. There is usually a failure of both input and output so that the person can neither read printed language nor indicate the meaning of a word spelled.

The degree of recovery from alexia is very variable. It is not uncommon for a rapid and complete recovery to take place, but, unfortunately, it is more common for recovery to be partial so that there is a limitation on the understanding of what is read. Sometimes there is no recovery at all. The degree of recovery largely depends on the level of literacy before the stroke.

WRITING

Writing difficulties are usually the result of right-sided paralysis in the right-handed, but damage to the back part of the brain, on the left side, can cause great difficulty in recalling the particular kind of movements needed to form letters on a page. A person may still be able, to spell a word given in speech, but will be unable to write it down. The disorder is complex and includes disturbance in the mechanical process of writing, loss of the ability to spell when writing, and difficulty in finding the correct word to write. Sometimes letters may be misplaced, omitted or reversed or a word may be written as an anagram or some letters repeated several times.

ARITHMETICAL SKILL

Sometimes a stroke affects arithmetical ability. This defect is usually associated with aphasia, but may, in rare cases be found on its own. This can be particularly distressing, for example, in the case of accountants who have had strokes, from which they have fully recovered except for the ability to handle numbers. One such unfortunate could not even accurately write down two-digit numbers dictated to him. Happily, when general recovery is good, the arithmetical facility will usually return, in time.

EFFECTS ON VISION

A considerable part of the extreme back of the brain is concerned with vision, and interruption of the blood supply by way of the vertebral arteries – the main source of blood to this part of the brain – will always affect vision. Visual loss from this cause is different from loss resulting from defects in the eyes. As in most cases of stroke, the brunt of the injury falls on one half of the brain and this produces a loss of vision in the corresponding halves of the field of vision of each eye. Nothing will be seen to one or other side of a central vertical line. Loss of half of the field of vision does not mean that there is a sort of black cloud covering half the field. This kind of visual loss is called 'hemianopia' and most patients have difficulty in describing it. Indeed they are frequently unaware of it and activities like driving are dangerous.

Differences between the two sides of the brain
For the great majority of people, the left half of the brain is the verbal or communication side. We have seen something of the effects of damage to this side but there are other differences between the two halves. The right side handles space relationships and our perception of them. This means the ability to appreciate the size and shape of objects and to judge their distance from us or each other. An artist with right-sided brain damage would still be able to manage the mechanical aspects of drawing or painting, but would produce seriously distorted work because of the inability to assess the relationship of the parts of the drawing.

The effect of this defect is much more widespread than this and activities like washing, eating, shaving, and so on, are likely to be made extremely difficult if the person concerned cannot tell right from left, or the inside of a garment from the outside, or the distance from a plate to the mouth. Strangely enough, the person with left-sided weakness often seems unaware of his difficulties and will usually attempt tasks beyond his ability, sometimes to his own, and others', danger. Also, because speech and communication are not affected it is easy to underestimate the difficulties and, perhaps, provide insufficient help. In contrast, the person with right-sided paralysis will go very slowly and clumsily and may be unable to communicate.

DEPRESSION AND OTHER PSYCHOLOGICAL UPSET

About a quarter of those who suffer a stroke develop depression due to brain damage. This is not simply the natural reaction to the catastrophe, although the effects of the two causes will overlap. True depression shows itself by a flattening of the mood so that there is no response to events which would normally give pleasure or satisfaction. There is also loss of appetite and weight, severe insomnia, failure of motivation and a general lowering of spirits.

There are several other very characteristic psychological responses usually caused by damage to brain function and it is important that they should be recognised as such. They are:

● Sudden emotional upset, with storms of weeping, which may be brought on by causes which would not normally have any effect on the emotions. These outbursts may have no relationship to the underlying mood of the person at the time and are clearly abnormal in nature.
● A tendency to swing suddenly from happiness to sadness and back again with little cause.
● A sense of hopelessness and a conviction that nothing can be done to help.
● A severe and disabling loss of confidence.

Stroke often leads to an apparent loss of intellectual ability. There may seem to be disturbance of the mental processes, with difficulty in grasping complex thought, and mild to severe loss of memory. I say 'apparent' because it is very difficult, in some cases, to be sure that these effects are the direct result of brain damage rather than the secondary effects of the person's awareness of, and emotional reaction to, what has happened.

This is especially true of loss of concentration and attention span and many of us would be affected in a similar way if we suffered severe disability without any question of brain damage.

Even so, genuine loss of memory and severe shortening of the attention span are common following a stroke and in many cases, they are due to actual disturbance of the relevant brain function. People affected in this way may seem childish, slow, irresponsible, lacking in interest in anything outside their own complaints and concerns and cut off from reality.

When memory is affected by stroke, matters which have been familiar for years tend to be retained much more strongly than recently acquired knowledge and this applies especially to things learned since the stroke. It is better, therefore, for the stroke patient to occupy familiar, rather than strange, surroundings and, when new skills have to be learned, these should always be based firmly on pre-existing knowledge.

PERSONALITY CHANGE

These psychological effects often seem to bring about a radical change in personality but it is difficult to assess how far this is due to actual brain damage. Often, the change is so obvious that brain damage must be assumed to be the cause. Personality change may be very hard to tolerate and may cause as much hardship to the spouse or carer as to the patient. The quiet, modest, reserved person may become loud and boastful; the shy recluse may become aggressively social and overtly sexual; the dominant personality may become submissive; the miser spendthrift, and so on. Often someone who formerly took a great pride in his appearance will become sloppy and will neglect personal hygiene. Happily, these changes can usually be corrected by patient guidance and re-education.

RECOVERY FROM STROKE

Sometimes recovery is almost total, sometimes slight, but, if the patient survives, some recovery almost always occurs. Most occurs in the first few weeks after the stroke; thereafter, progress tends to be slower. But recovery can, and does, continue for a very long time and proper management can increase the degree to which function is restored.

One of the most important of the many factors affecting recovery is age. This is well illustrated in the case of David who was lying in a deep coma, his breathing maintained by a mechanical air pump and his feeding provided by a permanent tube into his stomach. His parents were at his bedside, constantly talking to him in the hope of getting some sign of response. But as the weeks passed and he never made any voluntary movement, hope began to fade and the visits of his parents became less frequent. Only the physiotherapist seemed to believe that her devoted work to keep David's muscles from stiffening and contracting was worth the trouble. To my shame, I admit that I eventually concluded that the efforts to keep David alive were misguided.

Then one morning, to everyone's surprise, David began to move his arms and, progressively, over the next few weeks, his coma lightened and he began to respond to stimuli. But what kind of brain function could be expected after so much damage and such a long period of deep coma? David proved everyone wrong and recovered full consciousness and full awareness. Gradually his speech came back, not just the scanning, hesitant monotone so common in such cases, but a normal well-modulated voice expressing progressively more intelligent thought. After about four years no one, except those close to him could possibly have known of his previous condition.

This kind of story may not be of much comfort to the majority of stroke victims who do not have youth on their side. But *some* degree of recovery is the rule rather than the exception and observation of large numbers of older patients has shown that in many cases the degree of recovery is remarkable. These studies have also pointed to some important factors governing the extent of the recovery.

WHAT AFFECTS THE DEGREE OF RECOVERY?

- The more severe the stroke, the greater the long-term effect on behaviour and skills, and the longer the time needed for recovery.
- Strokes which come on gradually and progress slowly tend to cause less damage than sudden major strokes, and recovery from them will usually be better.
- Thoroughly learned and long-held skills are less likely to be lost or impaired than poorly or recently acquired abilities.
- People with high intelligence and strong character are likely to make a better recovery. People with emotional problems before the stroke will tend to make a less full recovery.
- Abilities acquired early in life will be less severely affected than those acquired later.
- The degree of recovery of function can be markedly affected by experience *after* the stroke.
- Treatment is much more effective in influencing the degree of

recovery if given sooner rather than later.

These last two points are especially important.

A natural disinclination to put any strain on the patient and a feeling that rest is necessary can have exactly the wrong effect. Stroke patients may have to be treated very firmly, even against their will if the fullest degree of recovery is to be achieved.

4 Learning to Walk Again

So far, we have looked at the theoretical background to stroke: how the brain works, its dependence on a good supply of blood, and the consequences of any interruption of that supply. Some readers may even have been able to profit by this information and take steps to reduce their own chances of suffering a stroke. But if you have a relative, husband or wife who has already suffered this misfortune, the matter is far from theoretical. It is now a major fact of life, involving distress, anxiety, social and perhaps economic disruption, and worrying alterations in relationships. Yet if nothing could be done to improve matters, this book would never have been written. The fact is that, given understanding and the correct approach to the various problems of the stroke victim, the functional ability and quality of life can often be greatly improved. As illustrated by the distressing case of Mrs Gowers, the failure to take proper action at the proper time, may, after the initial natural improvement, lead to a progressive worsening of the patient's state.

This chapter is mainly concerned with the means of restoring the fullest possible degree of mobility and, in suitable cases, normal walking. Obviously those who have suffered massive brain damage with widespread destruction of the nerves from the brain to the muscles, will never walk again. But even in these cases much may be done to improve their condition. It would be a fundamental mistake to assume, in any particular case, that the outlook is hopeless. Many wonderful recoveries have been achieved, but only in those who have been properly managed. Nature, left alone, will invariably produce a poorer functional result.

EARLY TREATMENT IS VITAL

The need for early intervention is well known to doctors and nurses dealing with stroke patients. Except for the gravely ill, all those treated in hospital will have the benefit of a good start in the management of their rehabilitation. But once patients are over the critical early stage and their condition has stabilised few hospitals can retain them. So responsibility inevitably falls on the patients, themselves, or on relatives, assisted by visiting nurses and, perhaps, physiotherapists.

Anyone faced with this kind of responsibility, whether to themselves or to another, may feel helpless and unhappy – perhaps even hopeless. Such a reaction is entirely natural and understandable. Despair over the future, severe depression, even terror, are the emotions common in this situation. But these are negative and destructive feelings which must be firmly put aside and replaced by constructive optimism based on knowledge of, and belief in, the correct management. The state of the mind powerfully affects the body. Positive, constructive thoughts actually do improve the condition and the abilities of the body.

Applying the principles in this book will not always be easy. There will be resistance, even resentment, and the task will be especially difficult if there are communication problems. But, somehow, cooperation and good motivation must be obtained if full success is to be achieved. If the reader is a stroke patient, then the mere fact that this book is being read suggests that motivation is already good. Perhaps even, if good advice has been obtained, a determined effort may already have been made to get out of bed and get the faculties working again. Cases like that of Mrs Gowers' occur only in the most exceptional and unusual circumstances. Even a minimal amount of common sense care, based on a few simple instructions, will prevent that sort of thing happening.

LYING IN BED IS DANGEROUS

The first aim in rehabilitation is to get out of bed. Most elderly readers, especially the more active, will be aware of the importance of maintaining physical activity if strength is to be retained. Three or four weeks in bed, from whatever cause, is a disaster for elderly people. Many never recover the strength they had before and those who do have to work long and hard. About one tenth of the remaining muscular strength is lost for each week spent at total rest. Even healthy young people take a longer period of time to return to full strength than the period they have spent in bed.

But the situation is positively dangerous with older people and it is no exaggeration to say that a fair number are actually killed by bed rest. Physical disuse causes rapid muscle wasting, not only to muscles paralysed by stroke, but also to the normal muscles. Softening and weakening of the bones from loss of calcium occurs and the danger of massive clots forming in the leg veins is considerable. These clots can come adrift and cause sudden death by embolism in the lungs.

So a first priority is the resumption of physical activity. In the very early stages, there will be a limit to this, although sometimes only by purely mental factors. The patient often feels sorry for himself and just wants to be left alone to lie in bed and feel resentful. In many cases the loss of body image, which is a consequence of the stroke, will add to the difficulty. A patient may actually feel that one side of his body does not belong to him and is of no concern, and in such cases it may be necessary to reinforce the awareness of the body by using mirrors.

A major additional danger concerns weight. An overweight stroke patient will be more sedentary than the average and will usually have a poor power-to-weight ratio. With reduced activity and, as the muscles begin to atrophy, the effective strength will very rapidly drop to the point where it is insufficient to allow recovery. Very fat people who suffer strokes – even quite minor strokes – are unlikely ever to walk again unless a supreme effort is made to get the weight down quickly. In addition overweight people may simply be too heavy for the helper to move so all sorts of problems will arise. These observations should persuade stroke victims of the importance of weight reduction. Immediate dieting is essential – nothing fancy or extreme, just eating a lot less than usual.

SPASM – THE ENEMY

Spasm is a subject of critical importance to all, especially to the stroke victim. Although it has already been introduced it is important to be clear what spasm is and how it comes about.

Damage in stroke occurs only in the brain and nothing at all has happened to the muscles themselves or to the nerves from the spinal cord to the muscles or those from the muscles to the cord. All these are intact and able to function. Even the connecting nerve bundles in the spinal cord are intact. The only thing wrong is that the nerve bundles passing down through the substance of the brain from the surface, whose job it is to tell the spinal nerves to stimulate the muscles into contraction, have been interfered with. The messages passing down from the brain surface – 'nerve impulses' – in addition to directing and initiating voluntary action, have a powerful controlling, smoothing and coordinating effect on the lower nerves running out of the spinal cord.

When the nerve impulses from the brain are absent, or abnormal, the lower nerves tend, after a time, to act on their own. But they cannot do this in a purposeful and smooth manner and the result is that the muscles affected are not only unable to perform voluntary actions but are also liable to go into uncontrollable contraction on the slightest stimulus. This condition, in which the muscles are unable to act under the control of the will, but readily contract in a purposeless manner, is called spastic paralysis and this is a very common feature of hemiplegia.

Almost all of the main muscle groups act in opposing pairs. For instance, the muscles which bend the elbow are opposed by the group which straighten it – but these opposing groups are not necessarily of equal strength. In order to stand upright and to walk, we have to fight gravity which would, without muscle contraction, cause us to collapse on to the ground. So the muscles which oppose gravity – those, for instance, which straighten the knees or bend the elbows – tend to be stronger than their opponents. Since spasm affects all muscles equally, the stronger ones will prevail and joints will be bent as a result of spasm of the anti-gravity muscles. This, in fact, is what happened to Mrs Gowers.

Positioning

This spasm must not be allowed to pull the body into an abnormal and fixed position of deformity. If it is not properly treated, an abnormal posture results and makes it impossible for the two sides of the body ever to be the same again. The head will flop over to the paralysed side. The hip, the knee and the ankle will be extended (just as they have to be to defy gravity) and the leg will rotate outwards. The elbow, wrist and fingers will be bent and the shoulder will be pulled backwards. So, right from the beginning, as soon as the patterns of spasticity begin to develop, the limbs *must* be positioned in such a way as to reduce the spasm. This is so, whether the person concerned is lying in bed, sitting up in a chair or even standing.

The positioning is done as follows: *The neck and spine must be straightened; the shoulder, on the affected side, must be raised; the elbow, wrist and fingers straightened, with the thumb held away from the hand and the palm facing outward; the leg must be held away from the body with the hip slightly bent and the foot turned upwards.* This kind of positioning must be adopted with the affected person lying, in turn, on the healthy side and on the paralysed side. If necessary, pillows must be used to keep the limbs in the appropriate position. Sitting up in a chair will help the positioning of the legs, but the affected arm must be supported on pillows to keep the shoulder elevated and the elbow extended. *It is particularly important to avoid a fixed bent deformity of the wrist and a 'cock-up' splint will often be necessary to achieve this.*

When the person is lying, the position greatly affects the amount of spasm. This is because information from all parts of the body is still being fed to the undamaged parts of the brain resulting in feedback which influences the amount of spasm. For instance, the position of the head has a great influence on the amount of spasm and if it is turned away from the paralysed side, spasm will increase. If turned towards the weak side, the spasm will be less. Because many stroke patients have a strong tendency to dissociate themselves from the paralysed side of their bodies – even to behave as if it did not exist – turning away is common and it must be actively resisted.

Lying on the back, except for short periods to relieve pressure discomfort, should be strongly discouraged. This is because it promotes spasm in the anti-gravity muscles and will quickly cause the body to take up the undesirable stroke position. If the patient does, briefly, lie on his back, great care must be taken to prevent abnormal positioning. A pillow should be put under the shoulder on the affected side to hold it forward and the arm must be pulled away from the body with the elbow straight and the wrist extended backwards. Likewise, the hip, on the paralysed side, must be propped forward with a pillow and the knee slightly bent with the foot resting on the bed and the paralysed knee on top of the other.

STARTING TO MOVE AGAIN

Movement should start as soon as no danger will result and certainly sooner rather than later. The first steps are to get the patient to roll over, sit up in bed and balance on the side of the bed. Until the patient is able to do these things alone, your help will be needed. The physiotherapist will advise here. Remember that the patient needs help on the *paralysed* side, so support should always be given from that side, rather than from the side which can support itself. This may sound obvious, but carers will often, thoughtlessly, support the good side.

Begin by practising rolling over, at first assisted, and then, as soon as possible, without assistance. The sooner the patient learns the trick of rolling on to either side, the sooner some measure of independence, however small, is achieved. This first exercise is not always as easy as it may seem. Rolling from the good side to the paralysed side is usually easy enough, but rolling on to the normal side from the weak side can be very difficult and requires a good deal of practice. The proper sequence is to clasp the hands together, with the arms extended and use the good arm to pull the paralysed arm straight up in the air, thus raising the weak shoulder. The head then turns to the good side and the extended arms follow, so that the balance of the body, assisted by the weight of the extended arms, begins to tip towards the sound side. The trunk, hips, legs and feet then follow round in turn.

When this sequence has been followed, the position which results is the correct anti-spasm one. Assistance with rolling over may be necessary, to begin with, but only the minimum of help should be given, and the aim should be to achieve active rolling, in both directions, without assistance, as quickly as possible. Because of the importance of the arm in positioning and rolling and because the arm on the weak side is, in a sense, a 'dead weight', there is a strong tendency for the shoulder joint on the affected side to suffer injury – even dislocation. This may easily happen, especially if the helper is unaware of the danger of inadequate support and of the risks of pulling on the paralysed arm. Special care must be taken of the weak arm during passive rolling movements and when dressing or moving the patient. As hemiplegia is often associated with sensory loss in the affected half of the body this may prevent the patient from being aware that the shoulder joint is being injured.

Some patients learn tricks to assist in rolling – for example, hooking the sound foot around the weak leg to assist the turn. But this encourages the patient to compensate for weakness by the use of the good side and simply promotes spasm in the paralysed side. Proper rehabilitation is therefore impeded. Loss of the muscle power on one side is often accompanied by loss of sensation so that the patient wants to ignore the paralysed side.

The carer must try to identify with the patient. Questions about what is being experienced must be asked. Remember that spasm is the enemy and any movement or position that brings it on must be avoided.

Even at this early stage the carer may feel that there is a major problem. The patient may be withdrawn and uncooperative, showing no sign of appreciation of what is being done and perhaps even actively resisting help. There may be outbursts of rage or inappropriate emotion and total lack of interest in the efforts made to improve functional ability. Every effort should be made to avoid discouragement. Any improvement achieved will not only give the patient hope, but will also make the carer's life easier.

Most stroke patients go through a stage in which they are extremely self-centred and, apparently unconcerned about the feelings of anyone but themselves. There are few exceptions to this and many responses may seem unkind or even cruel. But it would be wrong of you to react as one might to a person who has not suffered brain damage. Great patience is required and this is bound to fail at times.

SITTING UP IN BED

The first step towards getting out of bed is sitting up and learning sitting balance. Sense of balance will always be seriously impaired and it is important not to do too much at one time. The patient should not be left alone in a new position unless it can be maintained for a reasonable time and should sit well up in the bed, in a properly upright position and well supported by pillows so that the spine is not bent over to the weak side. The arm on the weak side must also be properly supported in the anti-spasm position. Remember that the elbow must be mainly straight, the shoulder forward, the arm rotated outwards so that the palm is upwards and the wrist extended backwards. The leg on the weak side must also be in the anti-spasm position – turned a little inward, the affected hip forward and slightly bent and the knee also a little bent and turned towards the midline of the body.

It is a basic mistake to assume that the bedside table should be placed on the patient's strong side. Although the spine should not be allowed to take up a permanent twist, by muscle spasm, to the weak side, it is nevertheless important that *active* voluntary movement to that side should be encouraged. This is best done by ensuring that the patient has to turn that way to reach the bedside table. This discourages spasm, encourages recognition of the affected side of the body and greatly assists rehabilitation. This automatically provides the motivation to move in the right direction. Very likely the patient will object, will want easy access and will want to ignore his affected side. The carer should explain the reasons and then be firm. But it is important to watch out for the position of the weak arm and ensure that it is not endangered in the process.

Working across the weak side is an important principle in the rehabilitation of a hemiplegic person and this point should be carefully noted. Pressure on the muscles of the weak side tell the brain that support is needed on that side and, as explained, this is mainly the job of the extra-pyramidal motor system. In a great many cases of hemiplegia, the extra-pyramidal system is still largely intact and it can supply the directions needed to the appropriate muscles which then contract in a purposeful manner. In other words, properly applied weight-bearing results in automatic support of the parts concerned. The same principle applies to walking.

GETTING OUT OF BED

Once sitting up in bed is achieved, no time should be lost in proceeding to get out of it. Again, the principle of working across the weak side is used. The patient will, therefore, have to get out of bed on the *paralysed* side and the first step is to learn how to prop up on the weak elbow and practice getting balance in this position while rolling far enough over to the edge of the bed to allow the good leg to cross over, and rest on top of, the weak leg. Although the eventual aim is to manage the whole business alone, the patient should not be allowed to go any further than this without assistance.

Having checked that the good leg is resting on top of the other, the carer should take a firm grip of the patient's good hand and, place the other hand behind the heel of the weak, lower, leg. By pulling gently on the hand and, at the same time, easing the legs over the edge of the bed and downward, the patient can be moved smoothly into a sitting position. As soon as this is done the position should be checked. Excitement over success must not lead the carer to forget the cardinal importance of proper positioning and the reason for correct positioning – to avoid spasm.

The feet should be placed firmly and flat on the floor, about eighteen inches apart and parallel to each other so that neither is turned in or out. This is important because the correct positioning of the feet ensure that the thigh is not allowed to rotate outwards – that is, to fall into the spasm position. The knees should be bent to a right angle, or as near as the height of the bed and of the patient will allow. If the bed is very high, some kind of stable low platform should be used.

With the arms stretched out sideways, so that the hands are on the bed, the patient should now be encouraged to begin shifting the weight from one haunch to the other and, as soon as this can be done, to begin shifting the body, by this alternating shift of weight, towards the edge of the bed and back again. The weight placed upon the weak arm in doing this will provide the stimulus necessary for reflex support. When this can be done satisfactorily, the fingers should be clasped together and the two arms held straight out in front while the haunch-walking continues. This provides excellent practice in balancing and in overcoming the natural tendency to fall to the affected side. Haunch-walking is also an aid to balance practice and should be done as vigorously as strength will allow. Try to get the patient to lift each hip clear of the bed, in turn.

These exercises are an important preliminary to relearning to walk, and should be done three or four times a day, or as often as the patient's strength will allow. Once haunch-walking has become easy, the next step is to get the patient up into a chair. A strong upright chair should be put alongside the bed with the edge of the seat on the patient's weak side. The patient should now be encouraged to lean on the good arm sufficiently to allow half standing, partial turning to the good side, and sitting down smoothly on the chair. The ability to do this without assistance is a boost to morale and a useful exercise.

Getting back into bed follows the same sequence in reverse, but involves the problem of raising the paralysed leg. At first assistance will be needed. Some patients learn to hook up the weak leg with the good one. This is certainly acceptable in an emergency and is an aid to independence, but it goes against the principle that all bodily movement should, if possible, be active. Passive movement – taking hold of a weak limb and moving it – may be useful, but it doesn't help in rehabilitation. Obviously a good deal of passive moving is necessary, especially in the early stages, but it is always a second best and deprives the patient of the opportunity to improve.

STANDING

The next stage is to get the patient to stand, and the method of doing this is also useful in getting back into bed. It is essential to understand the right way to do this before trying. This is how. The carer should ensure that the patient's feet are close together and should stand in front of him with the feet on either side of his. The carer's knees should be bent slightly so that they are positioned on either side of the patient's knees, and act as a sort of clamp for his. The carer is now in control of the patient's legs. The carer's hand is now put under the elbow of the patient's weak arm so that the forearm provides a rest for his. The carer can now lean over the patient a little and the patient puts his good arm round the carer's shoulders. The carer's arm is now put round the patient's waist.

This important position is more than just a way of raising a hemiplegic patient to his feet, or shifting him from a chair to a bed. It becomes almost a symbol of caring and provides confidence in standing and in weight-bearing on the affected side and is an essential stage towards unaided walking.

It will not, of course, be much good if the patient can stand only when held in this way, so some form of temporary support is needed. Two substantial chairs should be positioned on either side, seats outwards, with the backs level with the waist, and the patient should be persuaded to use the tops of the backs as 'parallel bars' for standing practice. Much persuasion should not be necessary if the patient has been sitting long, for the relief of standing is welcomed.

Now is the time for the patient to learn to stand up alone. This can be practised in several ways, but, at first, it is best to provide the support and confidence of the two chair backs. When used as an aid to standing up, the chairs should be placed reasonably close, one on either side, so that they do not tend to fall inward under the patient's weight. The two chairs should be placed just in front of the chair in which the patient is sitting so that the latter will have to lean forward a little with both arms stretched out to the parallel chair backs. These should be used only as a means of support and of maintaining balance while the patient stands up by leg and back power alone – not by dragging on the good arm. The exercise of rising to the feet and then resuming the sitting position should be repeated many times until strength and confidence have improved.

At this point it is very important to check that the spine is straight with the head held high and central. One thing that must be avoided at all costs is the common tendency to put all the weight on the good leg, so that the hip on the weak side is higher and the heel of the foot on the affected side off the ground. This, unfortunately, is the typical stance of the hemiplegic and once established may be difficult or impossible to correct. One out of three people who have had strokes and have progressed this far, develop this kind of stance and have, in consequence, a permanent and quite severe limp. The ankle becomes extended and only the ball of the foot rests on the ground. This condition may become permanent, with shortening of the tendon running down to the heel (the achilles tendon) and may be correctable, if at all, only by surgical operation. So attention should be paid to this, right from the beginning. The whole sole of the foot on the weak side must rest firmly on the ground and the hips must be level.

WALKING

The time at which walking should be started will vary from person to person, but, in any case, walking should always be preceeded by at least a week's daily standing and sitting practice. Longer than this will often be necessary. Skilled guidance in a physiotherapy department or rehabilitation centre is most important at this stage and should be arranged. It is natural to want to progress as rapidly as possible and care should be taken not to induce wrong habits which may be difficult to undo. If there is a delay in arranging proper physiotherapy, it may be best to limit the patient to sitting and standing exercises until professional advice can be obtained at a physiotherapy unit. In particular, crutches or a walking stick should not be used as these are likely to restrict the level of long-term success.

Walking is such a natural and unconscious activity to the healthy that one does not really appreciate what a complex process it is, and it is valuable to analyse what happens. The control of balance involves a great quantity of information being relayed to the brain from the eyes, the semicircular canals deep in the ears, the leg muscles and tendons and, indeed, every movable part of the body, and the integration of all that information by the brain to produce the appropriate signals to the muscles of locomotion. After stroke, a varying amount of this information may be denied and the integrating part of the brain may also have been damaged. So, quite apart from the one-sided weakness, balance itself may be defective and this may add to the difficulties. Fortunately, the brain is amazingly adaptive, even in the elderly, and, although some feedback information may be lost, the remaining sources can be called upon automatically to make good the deficit.

Walking involves forward momentum, the transfer of weight to one heel and then from that heel to the toe (with a lift which allows simultaneous swinging forward of the other leg), a firm push-off with the toe against the ground, to maintain the momentum, and then the repeat of the process on the other side. Obviously, a person with hemiplegia is not going to be able to carry out this process on both sides, but, so long as the weight can be borne on the affected side – making use of the extra-pyramidal system and reflex muscle contraction – and the foot can be flexed enough to allow the strong foot to come off the ground and swing to the front, momentum can be used to carry the body forward. In the ideal case a remarkably natural gait can be achieved.

Unfortunately many stroke patients are unable to bend the foot voluntarily and suffer a toe drop so that the toe scrapes along the ground during the swing forward. For these, a light leg caliper or brace may be necessary. This is attached to the shoe and has side pieces running up the leg to be strapped just below the knee. Whether or not a brace is necessary will be determined by the staff at the physiotherapy centre. The modern design is very inconspicuous and the brace is almost entirely concealed under the trousers or slacks.

In the early stages of walking practice at home, there will be a lot of anxiety about falling. This can be reduced by practising walking with a wall close to the weak side for any necessary support. The patient should not, however, rely on the wall and should move away as soon as confidence improves. If the hand on the weak side has a reasonable grasp, confidence can be improved by using a central walking balancing aid adapted from a sweeping brush with the handle shortened a little and a rubber tip pushed over the top of the handle. This should *not* be used as a walking stick or crutch but simply as an aid to balance. The ends of the head of the broom are held in two hands and the tip of the handle rests on the ground in front.

Above all, the patient should aim for naturalness in walking. Any limp or dip should be carefully scrutinised and investigated and, if possible, eliminated. This may not be easy, but the effort is well worth while. In re-learning to walk, the stroke patient actually makes use of the tendency to spasm – which if allowed to develop unchecked would probably make walking impossible. The object is not simply to drag oneself around somehow on two feet, but to do so in such a manner that no casual observer would suspect that there had ever been paralysis.

Walking sticks

If possible walking sticks should be avoided. When there is no other resource, a walking stick can certainly be a great help for balance and strength, but if used at an early stage might limit the degree of final recovery. In a sense, using a walking stick is an acknowledgement that the patient has decided to compensate for the weakness by using the normal side and has given up hope of improvement. When a long period has elapsed since the stroke, a walking stick may be a boon, but its correct use is not always well understood. This is dealt with, along with the use of other aids to mobility, in Chapter 8.

5 Psychology and Stroke

Our psychological state has a tremendous influence on our bodies – an influence which can hardly be exaggerated – and it operates continuously, gradually modifying the structure of our bodies, both in obvious ways, such as altering our bearing and carriage, and in more subtle ways of which we are much less aware until the evidence of bodily illness is forced upon us. A 'faulty' state of mind can, indirectly, lead to damage to the structure of our arteries, high blood pressure and stroke.

But the condition of the body also has a considerable bearing on the state of the mind and an event as major as a stroke will affect the mind profoundly. Because the brain is the seat of all mental activity, damage to its structure can also directly affect the mind. The consequences of these important points are dealt with in this chapter.

IS THERE A STROKE PERSONALITY?

The answer to this question is a very definite 'Yes'. Careful research has shown that some people, simply by the nature of their personalities, and the resulting behaviour patterns in their relations with others, are prone to illness. Anyone aware of stress and tension in their relationships or who suspect that their attitudes and responses may not be entirely healthy should certainly be taking precautions. Although it is probably impossible to make any really radical alteration in personality, it is not difficult to recognise the patterns of behaviour which are dangerous to health and which could lead to serious illness. Whenever possible, these patterns should be avoided or amended.

For at least twenty years, medical men have believed that among the small number of factors responsible for causing the changes in the arteries which lead to stroke or coronary thrombosis, one must include the possession of a particular type of personality. In one trial a group of over 3,000 men was divided into the high pressure, competitive go-getters (Type A personality) and the calm, relaxed, laid-back category (Type B personality). These men were then followed up for eight years and it was found that the Type A men had significantly more atherosclerosis than the Type B. Since coronary thrombosis is commoner in younger people than stroke, this was used as the index of artery disease and the early study showed that Type A people were twice as likely to have a heart attack as Type B people.

In more recent years critics of the theory have pointed out that it is often hard to identify these personality types with certainty and, although everyone recognises the extreme case, there are many who fall into neither category. Those who support the theory are able to give good descriptions of the Type A personality, and much research work has been done to try to improve the identification of a wider range of those at risk.

The Type A man (Type A women exist, but are less common than Type A men, and seem to be quite well protected against the undesirable effects) has a powerfully competitive nature with a constant sense of urgency and a determination to make the best use of his time. He does everything at top speed and tries to get through work as quickly as possible. He walks and drives quickly, always anxious to arrive and to get on with the next job. He talks rapidly and impatiently – often failing to finish sentences – and frequently interrupts. He has high motivation, is determined to succeed and, in the words of one of the originators of the concept, 'is aggressively involved in a chronic, incessant struggle to achieve more and more in less and less time.'

Careful studies on medical students and others have shown a fascinating correlation between the personality type and the amount of adrenaline and cortisol produced under stress. The medical students allowed the researchers to take blood samples as they were waiting, tense with anxiety, to go in to examinations. The results were clear. The type A people produced much higher levels of these hormones than the others. And we know that repeated high levels of these powerful substances tend to lead to arterial diseases – atherosclerosis and high blood pressure.

Hostility

The personality type theory has recently been refined even further by the discovery that the characteristic of the Type A personality most likely to be associated with atherosclerosis is *hostility*. Studies have shown that those people who demonstrate their competitiveness and impatience by strong hostility and indifference to the advantages and rights of others are in a very dangerous state. Personality can be reliably assessed by means of psychological tests, the best and most successful of these being the 'Minnesota Multiphasic Personality Inventory' (MMPI). This is a test in which the subject is asked to tick 'true' or 'false' to more than five hundred statements. From an analysis of the responses a remarkably detailed account of the personality of the subject can be obtained. The MMPI easily identified people with high hostility ratings. And when these people were followed up they had a mortality rate from arterial disease such as stroke or coronary thrombosis *six times as high* as those with low hostility ratings.

There are good physiological as well as psychological grounds for this remarkable finding. Unconcern for others often arises, in competitive people, from a feeling that if one does not protect oneself, others will take immediate advantage. Inevitably, this state of mind causes aggressive behaviour which, in turn, leads others to respond in the same way. This leads to anxiety and insecurity and, inevitably, further aggression. It also leads to stressful alienation and isolation. Distrust and fear of personal disadvantage, especially in a competitive context, means constant alertness – a state well known in the jungle and in the physiological laboratory. The need to be ready to fight or flee, at any moment, leads to the frequent production of adrenaline and cortisol and these hormones raise the blood pressure and increase the tendency of the blood to clot. Atherosclerosis, with the attendant risk of stroke or coronary thrombosis often results, in this indirect way, from such hostility.

Unquestionably, openly expressed hostility is dangerous – even speaking loudly for emotional reasons is known to raise the blood pressure, and plenty of people have suffered apoplexy in the heat of an angry tirade. But recent studies have now proved that when hostility is habitually bottled up, the effects on the health of the individual are often even more serious. A study of Type A men at Duke University, North Carolina, suggested that those who felt they should conceal their aggression against others and who succeeded, in spite of intense frustration, in avoiding a 'blow-up', were the ones most greatly at risk. Indeed, the research workers went so far as to suggest that this might be the only really important factor leading to a high risk of atherosclerosis and that it might have been the scattering of individuals of this particular characteristic within the Type A group that led to the higher than normal incidence of arterial disease.

This theory has yet to be proved, but if it is correct, the implications are important. Hard work, a sense of urgency and a determination to succeed may, it seems, be harmless so long as aggression is adequately controlled and, in particular, not 'bottled up'. We should all take a long, careful look at the nature of our relationships and the ways in which aggression is generated. Perhaps, if we understand how dangerous it can be to continue to live in such a way, we may be able to avoid it and spare ourselves the worst of the consequences.

MAKING THE PSYCHOLOGICAL ADJUSTMENT

The psychological effects of actually experiencing a stroke are well recognised and it is helpful if the carer is familiar with them so that the major events taking place in the mind of the victim can be understood. The mental response to suffering a stroke is essentially a grief reaction and the victim is actually mourning the loss of faculties and powers. At this stage the patient will not believe that recovery is likely, and part of the carer's job is to get this fact across, positively and effectively. Information of this kind is vital to the patient's mental security, but the carer will not be believed unless the statement is based on an authoritative source of medical information – such as this book.

Grief is the natural reaction to loss of any kind – of a person, money, a relationship or a faculty – and is a process of adaptation. It passes through a number of recognisable stages which are apparent to different degrees in different people. These include alarm, shock, denial, mitigation, anger, guilt, acceptance and adjustment. Not all of these may be recognised and often the stages overlap. Moreover, different people adjust at different speeds and the progress from one stage to the next is not smooth. This is likely to cause confusion and the behaviour of the patient may be very difficult to cope with. Help may, for instance, be rejected – especially if the patient is in the stage of anger, because everyone, including the carer, is likely to be blamed for what has happened.

In stroke, the significance of these phases is as follows:

● ALARM: this will be caused by the first TIA and may be severe. But, with repetition the level of alarm will drop and, eventually, the person may become almost indifferent to it. This is a great pity as early alarm of this kind can provide motivation for a change of lifestyle which could prevent stroke from occurring. Alarm at the time of the full stroke will be more severe, even intolerable, and will often be quickly followed by shock.

● SHOCK: this follows a full appreciation of what has happened and often acts as a kind of anaesthesia against the horrors of reality. The patient may show apparent indifference, perhaps even amusement – a sort of shock euphoria – and the carer must not be surprised at this or think that it is necessarily the result of brain damage. More likely it is the result of emotional damage and will probably pass into the stage of

- DENIAL: denial is an important defence mechanism used to reduce anxiety. It is not only employed by the patient but possibly also by the carer. Behaving as if very little had happened, avoiding talking about the patient's disability or anything connected with it, and engaging in a period of feverish activity with very little purpose are all signs of denial. But this mechanism has its function. It is a useful way of gaining time to come to terms with the problem and it will gradually pass. This may take longer for the patient than for the carer. Actively prolonging the period for the victim by reinforcing denial of the truth should be avoided. The carer should look out for indications of gradual acceptance and gently pursue the truth.

- MITIGATION: this phase need not occur but when it does it indicates an attempt to avoid the full distress of the situation by trying to make light of it. It is not a fully mature response and, if persisted in, will delay full acceptance and may undesirably postpone the acceptance of important early treatment.

- ANGER: this indicates the end of denial and the full realisation of the implications of what has happened. In many cases it passes fairly quickly but sometimes it persists to the great detriment of the patient. Anger will always be directed and, unfortunately, the carer may be the recipient. It is necessary to be very understanding and not to expect reason or logic when this powerful emotion is involved. Sometimes the anger is directed against God, and it is common, in this stage, for religious faith to be lost in a storm of bitterness against a Creator who could do such a thing. If religion has been an important element in the life of the sufferer, faith will probably be restored when the stage of resignation has been reached.

- GUILT: this may take various forms. Some people cannot accept that such a calamity could come upon them unless they deserved it. Stroke may be deemed by some to be a punishment and these people will experience guilt. Again, the stroke victim may feel that the family has been let down, possibly deprived of the standard of living they had come to expect. Commonly, the wife of a stroke patient will come to believe that she is responsible for what has happened by having driven him to work too hard. This is, of course, nonsense. Stroke is never caused by overwork and, in any case, it is doubtful whether anyone can ever be 'driven' to overwork. But if such guilt arises, and is accepted as justified, it may cause a reflected guilt in the mind of the patient, who is likely to be well aware that this is not the cause.

- ACCEPTANCE: this is the stage at which the stroke patient comes to terms with disability and, hopefully, begins to direct energy and

attention towards rehabilitation.
- ADJUSTMENT: after full acceptance a period of adjustment to the new situation occurs. So long as this adjustment is positive and constructive and is directed towards achieving maximal use of the remaining faculties, this is a healthy response.

These stages of reaction are a normal and, indeed, essential, part of the process of adaptation. To some extent they are protective and provide time for mental healing. So the carer should go along with them up to a point. But it is still necessary to see that the patient doesn't get stuck at one of the early stages. It is simply no good persistently denying what has happened, or cooperating in an insincere conspiracy to pretend that everything is going to be all right in the end. Reasoned optimism and a positive outlook, based upon known facts, are essential, but, as the truth gradually becomes apparent, it is important to acknowledge it openly.

MENTAL ATTITUDES IN RECOVERY

It is a basic mistake to think that the degree of recovery possible is entirely a matter of the degree of damage to the brain. Obviously this is an important factor, but it is by no means the only one. Different people with the same amount of brain damage may recover to remarkably different extents and many factors are involved. Some of these – such as the person's previous standard of health, the basic stability and flexibility of the personality, a generally optimistic outlook, the financial status and so on – cannot be controlled. But others can, and it is important to be aware of these.

The most influential mental factors are:

- The nature of the carer's attitude to the illness and to the patient's expectations of recovery.
- The extent to which the illness is understood both by the carer and the patient.
- The success with which the carer is able to maintain the patient's sense of continuing importance to others.
- The success with which the carer is able to keep up a meaningful relationship with the patient and maintain the patient's relationship with others.
- The success with which both carer and patient are able to keep emotions on an even keel.

These factors can make a great difference to the outcome. The victim must struggle, and will not do so unless there is a good reason. It is not uncommon for those with no motivation – and these are likely to be people who never had much inclination for life even before the stroke – just to turn their faces to the wall and wait for death. So it may be up to the carer to give the patient reasons to live – and one of the most effective of these is the belief that someone is genuinely concerned.

If, somehow, the carer has succeeded in really grasping what the patient is going through – in really getting inside the patient's mind – and if the patient understands this, then much will have been achieved. Failure in this will probably lead to misunderstanding, perhaps resentment and bitterness and even a permanent blighting of the relationship.

THE MIND OF THE VICTIM

Stroke is a devastating calamity, occurring usually when the person concerned has reached maximum earning capacity, and may have begun to look forward to the rewards of a lifetime's hard work. Instead, there may have to be a radical alteration in life-style, in social and economic status, earning power, future prospects and capacity for human relationships. Professional or business activities, which have been of absorbing interest – even of central concern – may have to be abandoned, and hobbies and sports may be impossible to pursue. Social activity may be seriously impeded and artistic and cultural interests cut off. Small wonder, then, that grave damage should be done to the mind of the victim and that the whole psychology should be altered for the worse. It is not surprising that stroke causes depression – sometimes suicidal depression.

Almost always, if the victim is a family man, he will have been secure in his position as head of the group. Even to those who do not often think about it, their status as undisputed leader and provider is an important one and the loss of this status is demoralising. Often it will be necessary for this role to be taken over by a wife or by some other member of the family and then decisions will be made which may not be to the satisfaction of the patient. Commonly, because the patient is unable to communicate, wrong assumptions are made about the degree to which he is able to understand what is going on. When this is so, frustration and anger may be extreme.

It is often assumed by relatives that apparently petty, child-like and hostile behaviour is just the result of brain damage. To some extent this may be so, but it should be remembered that much of the behaviour of the stroke patient is a perfectly natural response to what is an intolerably painful situation. And if, instead of sympathetic understanding, there is resentment by the family – at lowered income and the need to do menial tasks for the patient – and his resentment is reflected in the attitude, then a very unhappy state of affairs is inevitable – one in which the patient will react with opposition, complaint and even savage aggression.

DEPRESSION

Depression is easily understood and is usually a reaction to the circumstances. The feeling of uselessness, the loss of self-esteem, the frustrations and the inability to communicate, inevitably lead to depression. Depression is especially common in those people who remain in full possession of their mental faculties but who are unable to speak or communicate in other ways. And it is more likely to affect those who, before the stroke, were of a gloomy and pessimistic nature than those who had a naturally cheerful disposition.

When depression is a natural consequence of the patient's awareness of the catastrophe, it is called 'reactive depression' and it is identical to what would happen to someone who had not suffered a stroke but who had to put up with the same degree of life damage. Because the damage to the brain functions is always greatest at the onset, depression does not usually start immediately after the stroke, but generally comes on several weeks, or even months, later. If it does not occur at all then it is a rather bad sign, because it suggests that the patient does not really understand what is happening. Obviously, a person who shows reactive depression to a stroke has retained considerable intellectual power. So, although it is upsetting to the relatives, it should be regarded as an encouraging sign, indicating that the essential function of understanding is largely unimpaired.

Depression shows itself in a number of ways. Commonly, the patient seems to turn inwards and give up all attempts at communication. There may be refusal to listen even when matters of great importance are being discussed. There may be a general failure of cooperation, even in such things as eating and excretion, and, in particular, there may be an unwillingness to go along with attempts at rehabilitation.

If there is a strong element of frustration associated with the depression, the effect may be very serious and attempts at suicide are not unknown in such cases. Well-meaning and persistent attempts to try to force the patient to perform tasks which were formerly easy, but are now almost too difficult, may lead to gathering frustration, resentment and anger and a profound depression. This situation may progress to an emotional crisis – what used to be called a 'nervous breakdown' – with weeping and aggression and an obvious wish for total withdrawal from the humiliating demands of the would-be helper. This kind of acute breakdown of motivation will usually last for only a few hours but may, occasionally, last for days. Ideally, such crises should not occur and when they do, there is a clear indication of a failure of communication.

Persistent depression can interfere seriously with rehabilitation and along with fear, a sense of hopelessness and a lack of purpose, should be avoided, or strongly combatted, if possible. Negative outlook is fostered largely by faulty attitudes in those looking after the patient. Stroke patients usually understand much more than they are able to indicate and can think much more clearly than one would infer from their behaviour. An appreciation of this and a determination to allow them to do as much as they can for themselves and, indeed, to exercise as much control as possible over their own affairs, is the surest means of combating depression.

EMOTIONAL UPS AND DOWNS

It is difficult to know how far emotional instability, which is so common after stroke, is simply a reaction to the disaster – a perfectly normal grief response to the loss of life-quality – or how far it is caused by brain damage. Stroke patients weep a lot but some also laugh more than is appropriate. Crying, in response to a reminder of what one was, or was once capable of, is probably a normal response. But inappropriate tearfulness or laughter indicates a disorder – possibly quite minor – of brain function. Fortunately, emotional instability usually clears up completely within a few months. But while it is present it can be distressing or annoying and serves no useful purpose. Try to stop a display of inappropriate emotion by directing the patient's attention elsewhere. This works well.

The effects of stroke are so complex that one cannot always be sure that the emotion displayed is actually being felt. The patient may show all the signs of enjoyment while being miserable, or manifest furious anger while not actually being angry at all. The signs of emotion are usually taken at face value and it is very difficult not to react to them in the normal way. This is especially so with emotions such as anger which seem to threaten us. So, unless unusual patience and forebearance are shown, there will always be misunderstanding and unnecessary trouble. To someone trying only to help, an aggressive response is always painful.

The situation is not helped if the spouse – usually a wife – thinks that she is guilty of bringing about her husband's stroke by her demands – financial, social, even sexual. This is a common reaction among the wives of hard-working, successful men who suffer strokes. Such a reaction is understandable but illogical. Strokes are not caused by hard work, but by a basically defective personality, a lifetime of self-abuse by dietary over-indulgence, inadequate exercise and smoking, and by the inheritance of genes predisposing to cardiovascular disease. The tendency to build up stress by engaging in high-pressure, competitive work is not likely to be the result of a wife's urging, but will almost always be a constitutional quality.

Hostility to other people, especially if constantly repressed, is, as we have seen, a stress factor predisposing to arterial disease, but even if a wife recognises that this might have been the cause of her husband's illness, she can hardly blame herself for that.

Worry about Sex

A major cause of mental upset is the fear of the loss of sexual ability. Often, this fear is without foundation, as many who have suffered even quite severe strokes remain physically capable of effective sexual performance. But sexual ability is so sensitively affected by the state of mind that a stroke is almost bound to diminish sexual power through its damaging effect on the patient's own sense of physical and social worth. Once this mechanism is understood, confidence in sexual capacity may begin to be restored.

This important subject is dealt with in Chapter 7.

Legal responsibility

This is a very difficult problem and one which may cause much unhappiness. The stroke victim may be a person of wealth or influence, accustomed to wielding power. Major questions may arise when such a person is thought to be no longer competent to discharge legal rights responsibly. The extent to which speech can be understood and rational decisions made are often questioned in such cases. Inability to recall the names of objects or people or to express any concept in words, often leads to a strong presumption of lack of the necessary legal responsibility to manage personal and family affairs. It is very difficult to assess the intelligence of a person when the usual routes of communication are blocked.

But it is important to remember that most stroke patients who are aphasic understand much more than they are able to show, and have a greater ability to think than is apparent. The inability to communicate does not mean that nothing is going on inside the patient's head. Indeed, many stroke patients who are almost completely uncommunicative are experiencing a rich, if somewhat depressing, intellectual life. Should one fail to appreciate this, and act towards such patients as if they were mentally defective, the result will be a deepening of the depression and a tremendous impulse to hostility.

So stroke patients should always be given the benefit of the doubt and should be assumed, until it is proved otherwise, to be capable of normal mental activity. Of course, experience may show that this is not so. If decisions are made which are obviously at variance with common sense, there are grounds for suspecting that the patient may not have legal competence. But one must be extremely careful not to reach a conclusion on inadequate grounds.

Many stroke victims, even those with severe aphasia, are perfectly capable of managing their own affairs, and are entitled to do so. When questions of inheritance arise, disappointed relatives, aware of the contents of a new will, may be tempted to seek a remedy in trying to have the testator declared legally incompetent. In this event, the stroke victim is entitled, at the very least, to skilled medical and psychiatric assessment, and proper legal representation, before a decision is made.

6 Problems of Communication

Sense shut in

The door of my consulting room was open and the nurse outside was talking to the patient as one might talk to a small child. When he was wheeled in his face was working and he was trying to speak.

'A-ab . . . a-ab, yes, a-ab . . .' was all he could manage.

I don't know what was in his mind but I knew that the Commander was a cultivated and educated man, that his intelligence was unimpaired, his memory barely affected and his interest in scientific and artistic matters keen.

The nurse was a kindly, sensible girl who would normally have been entirely respectful. Yet, talking in a slow, loud voice, as if he were deaf, and using language appropriate to someone with a mental age of about four, she had been going on about what a naughty boy he was to let his right hand fall into the spokes of the wheel-chair. I wondered if he were choking with rage inside, or whether he had now learned to accept this kind of thing philosophically . . . To get the message across to the nurse indirectly I started to talk to the Commander about the disaster of the space shuttle explosion. He listened intently, his eyes fixed on my face, and nodded appropriately. It was clear that he was grateful.

Why do we treat stroke patients in this way? The nurse's attitude was obviously determined by the extent to which the patient could communicate with her. Although people's appearances influence us a good deal, it is essentially the quality of their minds which cause us to react to them in a particular way. But if their minds have no ready access to us, we are apt to treat them as if they were mindless. The Commander, deprived of his habitual channels of communication – speech and facial expression – existed for the nurse only as a rather clumsy and helpless individual, who could not even thank her for what she was doing for him. He could write, but being paralysed in his right side, he had to depend on his left hand and writing was very awkward.

The nurse was well aware that many stroke patients have suffered much more serious functional damage than just one-sided paralysis and loss of the ability to speak. She knew that many also have a severe defect of understanding and that some of them, although able to talk freely and fluently, don't make any sense. She knew that many stroke patients are irritable and bad-tempered, many are withdrawn and uncommunicative, even if they are able to speak, and that many are so wrapped up in their own distress and resentment that they can't concern themselves with anything else. What she had not perceived was that, frequently, this kind of behaviour is precisely the sort of response one would expect from someone who is being treated in an inappropriate manner and who is incapable of pointing this out. Perhaps it was because she had so often had to deal with patients with whom no sort of communication was possible that she tended to treat them all in this way.

THE CAUSE OF APHASIA

About one stroke patient in three suffers some damage to the function of communication, particularly if the right side of the body is paralysed. The right side of the body is controlled by the left side of the brain and it is in the left half of the brain that the power of speech, and all the other faculties concerned with communication, are normally situated. So cerebral ischaemia or haemorrhage involving the right half of the brain produces a weakness of the left side of the body but would not normally affect speech. In a very small number of left-handed people, the right half of the brain is dominant and if such a person had damage to the right half of the brain, speech would probably be affected.

The Commander's case was a little unusual in that the damage to the speech area in the left side of his brain was confined to a comparatively small segment concerned only with the mechanical aspects of speech. He knew exactly what he wanted to say, and the precise words with which he wished to express his thoughts; his ideas were fluid and appropriate and sometimes they were bursting to get out. But when he tried to speak, the only sounds he could make were meaningless noises. He was a quick-minded man who had been capable of clear and effective expression and suffered great frustration in trying to converse by such means as playing 'Twenty questions'. I had watched him practising left-handed typing on a portable micro-computer with a word processor program, to improve his communication.

The Commander had actually suffered more subtle damage than simply one-sided paralysis and loss of the power of speech. Examination showed that if, having covered his eyes, I moved one of his fingers or toes passively into a new position, he would be completely unable to say in which direction it had been moved. Likewise, if a small object, such as a coin, were put into his hand and he was encouraged to try to identify it by feel, he would be unable to do so. Happily, with the passage of time, and by dint of sheer, stubborn determination, the Commander mastered his word processor (although he always had to look at his fingers when typing) and is now writing a book on Naval Intelligence in World War II.

TYPES OF SPEECH DEFECT

Speech defects are a little more complex than so far indicated and the speech centre can suffer various types of damage. In the most general terms, speech defect can be divided into two categories. On the one hand, there may be a defect in the ability to understand speech, so that normal expression is impossible. On the other hand, although understanding may be perfectly normal, the central control of the breath, the mouth cavity, and lip and tongue movement, may be defective so that the coordination necessary for normal speech is impossible. Quite apart from these defects, the muscles used for speech may be weak. Paralysis of one side of the face is very common in stroke and, inevitably, the muscles around the mouth will be affected causing slurred, puffy speech. This kind of speech defect is basically different from that caused by a defect of the central, nervous control of the function of speech.

There may be loss of the ability to name familiar objects or to understand the meaning of words. There may be actual word deafness, or loss of the power to string words meaningfully together, so that speech becomes a sequence of unrelated words. The patient may be unable to originate speech but may be able to repeat words spoken by others. Worst of all, there may be a total loss of all the communication functions, so that the patient neither takes in nor gives out any information. This is a tragic situation in which the individual is, so far as we can judge, wholly cut off from the outside world. There is no way of knowing what such an experience can be like, but there may be some comfort in the thought that, in all probability, there is a dampening of consciousness so that suffering is minimised. Those who recover from such a situation seldom have much recollection of what it was like.

ASSESSING THE DAMAGE

It is important for a relative or spouse of a stroke patient to find out as soon as possible what is going on inside the patient's mind. A realistic assessment of the severity of the damage must be made to discover how much insight the patient has into the situation. To this end, effective communication, if this is at all possible, is vital. A failure of communication will be a disaster, both for the patient and for the carer. Understanding what the stroke victim is going through, identifying, and, above all, trying to make sure that the carer's concern is understood, will do more for morale and motivation towards recovery than almost anything else.

Effective communication may take some time and it may be difficult to decide how much success is being achieved. The carer should prepare for the worst but act as if assuming the best. There should be no baby talk and no patronising attitudes. Normal behaviour – talking normally about normal subjects and about the illness – is best. Deliberate, slowish speech, without shouting is helpful. Short sentences with pauses will give time for assimilation. But, as soon as possible, the carer should try to establish whether or not this is necessary.

A channel of communication must be established as soon as possible – a 'yes or no' code of nods, head shakes, hand pressure, etc. – and tested regularly. If, at first, there are inconsistencies, these may well resolve in time. For instance, the patient may, initially, signal, or say, 'yes' when 'no' is meant, and may not even be aware of it. But the probability is that the patient *is* aware of the error, and signs of severe frustration and annoyance may be evident. The majority of stroke patients get back a considerable faculty of speech but the degree of recovery is very variable and the recovery phase may be a period of grave hardship.

Some of the effects of stroke are obvious – the inability to move one side of the body, the loss of feeling in the skin, the loss of speech function, the incontinence, and so on. But other effects are more subtle and tend to be concealed and it is important that the carer should be aware of the more important of these. Indeed, it is only the carer who is likely to be in a position fully to assess the change. A relative will have more time to devote than medical staff and will probably be able to find out a lot more than the doctor. Even more important, the trouble taken in doing so will mean a great deal to the sufferer. Patient and careful investigation will be necessary, but the trouble is likely to be rewarded.

However, attempts to assess the situation should not humilate or embarrass the patient. The attempts should be private and should be clearly explained. As soon as something has been learnt of the state of the person's mind, reactions should be adjusted accordingly. The patient must not be forced to respond to trivial tests over again as this will serve no useful purpose and will only annoy.

Apart from speech function, other things to consider are:

- The state of the reasoning power
- The state of the memory
- The ability to recognise or name objects
- The awareness of the function of objects
- The ability to read and to understand what is read
- The ability to write

The loss of the ability to perform learned physical skills, such as writing, may be quite independent of physical paralysis. Paralysis will make certain actions impossible, but stroke can deprive the patient of skills – such as brushing the teeth, playing a musical instrument, driving, etc, – even if the muscles used for these skills are still capable of functioning.

HOW TO ASSESS THE MENTAL CAPABILITIES

As speech defect can be, and often is, entirely independent of any change in the mental status it must not be assumed that because the patient can no longer talk there has necessarily been some mental deterioration. But it is important to try to find out. Hasty conclusions must be avoided. A clear distinction should be made between memory loss and loss of reasoning power and remember that the ability to name or recognise objects can be damaged by stroke although the mental powers, in the broader sense, may be entirely unimpaired.

When the channel of communication has been made, it should be explained that, to discover the extent of the damage caused by the stroke, some tests are necessary. The patient should be asked if there is any objection. If the intellectual powers are unimpaired the patient will greatly welcome the chance to show it. If the mental powers are severely diminished, this suggestion will not be understood and is unlikely to cause distress. The test is so arranged that questions can be answered by using a 'yes' or 'no' code, but if the patient can write, this will make things much easier. Even if only left-handed writing is possible this may be better than using a code. The test should be worked through slowly and conscientiously and a careful score kept. It may be repeated at intervals of several weeks to check progress of recovery. The following is a suggestion of the sort of questions to ask but these can be varied in accordance with the patient's previous knowledge.

Test of higher brain functions
Each correct response scores four points. Errors score nothing.

1 Is the present Prime Minister called Churchill, Eden, Macmillan, Wilson, Heath, Callaghan, Thatcher?
2 What year is it? (Start five years back)
3 Is it Summer, Autumn, Winter or Spring?
4 Is it morning, afternoon or evening?
5 Take 7 away from 93. Is the answer 90, 89, 87, 86 or 85?
6 Take 7 away from 51. Is the answer 47, 46, 45, 44 or 43?
7 What town/village are we in? (Give five alternatives, four wrong.)
8 What street are we in? (Give five alternatives, four wrong.)
9 What is the house number? (Give five alternatives, four wrong.)
10 Are you downstairs?

Get together a watch, a ball-pen, a pencil, a ruler, a table knife and a book. Hold up each in turn.

11 Is this a knife? (Score for correct answer of 'no')
12 Is this a ruler?
13 Is this a pencil?
14 Is this a watch?
15 Is this a ball-pen?
16 Is this a book?

Hold up the watch.
17 Is this for writing with?

Hold up the ball-pen.
18 Is this for cutting with?

Hold up the pencil.
19 Is this for writing with?

Hold up the ruler.
20 Is this for telling the time?

Hold up the knife.
21 Is this for reading?

Hold up the book.
22 Is this for drawing lines with?

23 What is your name? (Give five alternatives, four wrong.)
24 What is my name? (Give five alternatives, four wrong.)
25 How do you think you have done in the test? Well? So-so? Badly?

It would be wrong to think that this kind of test gives more than a rough indication of the percentage of damage to brain function, but it will tell you a great deal about the specific *nature* of the damage. A score of 100 indicates that the stroke has not affected orientation in time and space, has not grossly disturbed the reasoning power, and has had no severe effect on the memory. Don't be unduly disturbed by a low score. Remember that progress and gradual improvement are the rule rather than the exception. And remember, too, that a person recovering from stroke will have good days and off days, so that performance may, at first, vary quite a lot. The test should not be done too often despite the anxiety of the carer.

The response to tests of this kind will help you to avoid the kind of unthinking and ill-informed impatience so often shown to stroke victims by those who don't really understand what is going on.

Unfortunately, many stroke patients will be unable to cooperate in the testing in the early stages but a patient who is mute and unresponsive soon after the stroke may, some months later, be back at work apparently in full possession of all faculties, and the extent of improvement gained by the right kind of rehabilitation procedures is dramatic.

RESTORATION OF SPEECH

This is a major task, but one in which the devotion, love and patience of a carer or partner can be amply shown. It is not a job to be undertaken without skilled supervision and the primary responsibility for the management rests with the speech therapist who should be involved at the earliest possible stage. The success of speech therapy depends more on the patient, and on the severity of the damage, than on the knowledge and skill of the therapist and there are, regrettably, cases in which even the most devoted care will lead to nothing. But if the potential for recovery is there, the degree of success will depend considerably on the therapist and the carer.

A good therapist will be aware of the vitally important role the concerned partner can play in bringing about maximal recovery, and will always try to involve relatives and friends in the process. But it should be understood that, even under the best circumstances, recovery will inevitably be slow.

FACTORS AFFECTING RECOVERY_____

The older the patient at the time of the stroke, the worse the outlook. The level of intelligence, literacy and, to some extent, education will also affect the outcome. The inevitable anxiety and depression after a stroke will lead to lack of concentration and thus impede recovery. Damage to other brain functions – memory loss, disorientation, visual disturbances, giddiness, and so on, will impose more problems and make the outlook proportionately worse. Impairment of understanding will reduce communication with the speech therapist but if therapy is delayed until a late stage, it is likely to be much less successful.

Natural recovery
In a great majority of cases, at least some degree of spontaneous recovery of the faculty of speech may be expected. Most of the natural recovery takes place in the first four or five weeks and any recovery enjoyed after that is due largely to speech therapy. This may be true even if no formal therapy is provided. It has been found that many stroke patients, determined to communicate again, actually develop new ways of conveying information to others and that this activity contributes to recovery. One of the most important elements in promoting recovery is the patient's morale. Indeed, some experts have suggested that the *whole* benefit from speech therapy comes from the improvement in patient motivation resulting from devoted attention.

Whether this is true or not, there is every reason to believe that if the patient thinks that the work being done is half-hearted, casual or uncaring, there is unlikely to be much benefit from it. So it is important for those in contact with a stroke victim to maintain an attitude of expectant optimism and encouragement.

HOW TO ACT TOWARDS AN APHASIC PERSON_____

Aphasia has nothing to do with mental defect and patronising attitudes are deplorable. The carer should try to be normal at all times but it will probably be greatly appreciated if speech is a little slower than usual, with clear expression and simple language. Too much should not be put into one sentence – many aphasic people are easily confused by complexity. Time must be allowed for ideas to be assimilated. Every channel of access must be used. The carer should always supplement expression by gesture or any other available means. If the written word is more easily understood than speech, or if writing proves to be an aid to comprehension, then this should be used to communicate, however slow and tedious this may be.

When the patient is struggling for words, there is a strong temptation to finish sentences. This should be avoided – the patient is as much concerned with getting the word out as with conveying meaning. The approach should be natural with respect for the patient's dignity.

Aphasia from the patient's point of view

One of the most common problems the aphasic person will have is a simple inability to find the right word. Remember how frustrating it is for someone who is not aphasic to try to recall a name, and then imagine what it must be like to have this problem for the majority, or even all, of the words you need. What the aphasic person has to do is to hunt for another word with the same meaning or to talk around it and find, if possible, an alternative way of expressing the same thing. This may be very difficult but the attempt must be made.

Even worse than this universal forgetfulness is the difficulty of producing the names of well-known objects. An aphasic may look at a telephone and be perfectly well aware of what it is used for – may be perfectly capable of using it correctly – but may be totally unable to associate the object with the word 'telephone'. If asked what it is called, the response may be: 'It's for calling Michael.' Even when a mental concept of the word can be formed, there may then be the additional difficulty of articulation.

Memory loss is not confined to words. All sorts of data may be submerged – it is unlikely that data has actually been destroyed. In all likelihood the information is still present and there is always the chance that access will be restored. Information stored recently is much more likely to be inaccessible than long–held data. This is because material which has been stored for a long time will usually have been repeatedly recalled and used, and we know that this is the best way to improve the accessibility of stored information. An important consequence of this fact is that it is unkind to shift a stroke victim away from a familiar environment as this may cause great difficulty. The right place for a recovering stroke victim is at home, in familiar surroundings and associations and visited frequently by well-known friends.

METHODS OF SPEECH TRAINING

Although the carer can do a great deal to help with speech training, and is in many ways the most important member of the team, the professional speech therapist has an essential part to play. Her first job is to make a detailed assessment of the degree of the defect and of the extent to which speech is affected by involvement of the muscles of the lips and tongue (dysarthria) as well as the speech and comprehension centres in the brain (expressive and receptive dysphasia). Having made this analysis, it is very important for the speech therapist – and this is something all speech therapists recognise – to ensure that friends and relatives, and especially the person chiefly responsible, are fully briefed on the particular difficulties and are then guided in the best way to proceed with the training.

Unfortunately, the therapist may decide that very little can be done. But even among those deemed least likely to recover, a remarkable degree of restoration of speech has occasionally occurred. One should never be too pessimistic – the trend, in almost all cases, is towards gradual recovery and this may continue for weeks or months. A continuous improvement, should not, however be expected. More often, recovery seems to occur in jumps, with long periods when little improvement seems to be taking place. It is important to maintain an attitude of confident optimism. This may be very difficult in the face of little apparent progress, but it may be essential in maintaining the patient's motivation.

Communication problems often involve more than just speech difficulty. If language comprehension is severely affected this will, of course, make training additionally difficult. Happily, studies have shown that a defect of speech understanding is the problem most likely to resolve spontaneously, so this should not be allowed to cause too much discouragement.

Many different approaches to speech re-training have been developed and most of these have had some success. Approach varies from patient to patient and some experimentation may be desirable. Each case is unique and must be given individual attention, dictated by the therapist.

One very promising method of speech re-training is MIT – 'melodic intonation therapy'. The idea is based on the observation that some severely aphasic people, quite unable to speak a particular word or phrase, are able to sing it. Musical skills originate in the right half of the brain and, of course, aphasic people almost always have a defect in the left half. The therapist gets the patient to sing short phrases in imitation of her own performance, and then gradually increases the length and complexity of these phrases. No particular sense of musical pitch is required and some very odd droning noises come from some patients, with excellent effect.

An additional technique used in the MIT system makes use of the characteristic rhythm of the phrases being tried. As the therapist speaks or sings a particular phrase in a clear and rhythmical manner, the patient taps out the rhythm with a pencil. This precise rhythmical pattern is then repeated frequently by the patient, while tapping, and at the same time attempts are made to speak the phrase. The method depends on the principle that the sound of the rhythm, and even the movement of the hand to achieve the tapping, provide information about the phrase – clues which are often sufficient to make the difference between failure to speak at all and the ability to articulate. Once the phrase can be sung, and then spoken, with the tapping, the latter is gradually withdrawn and eventually spontaneous speech becomes possible.

MIT has been used all over the world to help patients and has often been very successful but it is not of value in all cases of aphasia. Those best helped, as might be expected, are the people whose comprehension is well preserved and whose problem is essentially one of producing the required sounds and rhythms.

All methods try to make use of various avenues of communication. For instance, an attempt to understand speech will often be more successful if the spoken words are accompanied by successive pointing to the same words in print or writing, or to a relevant picture. It is *not* a good idea to try to convey the sense of words *one at a time* or to encourage the speaking of single words. Short phrases are always better. Another channel of communication which has proved valuable as an aid to recovery is sign language. There are several sign languages and all can be useful. Although a person who had a left-brain stroke with speech defect will usually also have problems in using a sign language, trials have shown that some patients make real progress in restoring speech by using this method.

The more elaborate sign languages are often about as difficult to use as natural language, but one particular system, derived from the North American plains Indians and called 'Amerind' has proved very useful both as an aid to recovery and as a practical aid to communication. Amerind can be done with one hand only – a very useful feature for people with hemiplegia – and is very simple with quite a small number of different signs. The meaning of most of them is fairly obvious and about three-quarters of them can be understood without explanation – or at least can be understood by non-aphasic people. Obviously, if Amerind is going to be used as a substitute for speech, it will have to be learned by the carer and other members of the family as well as by the patient.

Experience with the use of sign language has led workers to consider whether other methods of non-verbal communication could be useful. If the affected person can be made to learn the meaning of a range of abstract symbols which can be printed on cards or embossed on plastic discs, then communication will be possible simply by presenting these symbols. Oddly enough this idea started with attempts to communicate with chimpanzees using symbols – attempts which were encouragingly successful. It has been shown that patients with severe aphasia, both expressive and receptive, can learn to use such a system to communicate.

Psychotherapy for aphasia

Stroke victims have major problems which no one could be expected to cope with in a state of relaxed emotion. Proper motivation is important in promoting recovery and control over the emotions is essential. The disturbance of the language function, alone, is enough to cause a major psychological upset, for speech and human communication are central to our human emotional needs. Except in certain rare cases where brain damage has led to an abnormal lightening of the mood, depression is an almost universal feature of the early weeks of the aphasic.

Unfortunately, conventional psychotherapy involves much verbal inter-action between the patient and the doctor, with the patient doing nearly all the talking, and this, of course, is the very thing the aphasic patient can't do. Frustratingly, the aphasic person is longing desperately to make others understand what it is like to be cut off, in this way. For those capable of some degree of communication, however small, psycho-therapy, especially in the form of group therapy, can be valuable in a number of ways. The opportunity to express, to a receptive and understanding person or group, the distress and the problems facing one, is, in itself, therapeutic.

Participating in group discussion, so far as possible under the guidance of a skilled psychotherapist, can bring several advantages. Some patients have discovered that a major part of their difficulty in communicating was due to unjustified anxiety that others would not understand them. Group therapy has enabled many to overcome the natural fear of making fools of themselves – a fear which had previously been severely inhibiting.

Drugs acting on the emotions ('tranquillisers') do not have a very large part to play in the treatment of aphasia, although if prescribed selectively by an expert, and used over a relatively short period, some can help by relieving anxiety and depression and promoting a mood of optimism.

Other people's experience

Some people who have returned to a varying degree of normality have been prompted to give others the benefit of their experience. These people write with impressive courage and determination and should be a source of inspiration and motivation to sufferers. Here is a short list of titles, with authors and publishers:

Learning To Speak Again After a Stroke Charles R. Isted (King Edward's Hospital Fund for London, 1979)

A Stroke in the Family Valerie Eaton Griffith (Wildwood House Ltd, 1975)

Stroke – Who Cares? Pauline Willis (Turner-Lord Publications, PO Box 171, Vaucluse, New South Wales 2030, Australia, 1985) (Mrs Willis writes about her experience as a carer.)

Stroke' A Diary of Recovery Douglas Ritchie (Faber and Faber, 1966)

Postscript from a Patient J.A.S. MacDonald, in *Restoration of Motor Function in the Stroke Patient* (Churchill Livingstone, 1983)

Some of these books are described more fully at the end of Chapter 10.

7 Stroke and The Sex Life

Sexuality is such a deep-rooted element in human biology that it affects all our relationships, intimate or otherwise. In close human associations, satisfactory mutual sexual expression leads to confidence, happiness and contentment. 'Sexual expression' does not simply mean physical sexual intercourse, but includes all the effects of the partners' awareness of the physical, mental and emotional differences between them. The sexual act itself is, or should be, an 'expression' or demonstration of the feelings of love, appreciation, gratitude and solidarity experienced by the partners. In younger people, the purely erotic and sensory element may assume an overwhelming importance, but in a mature relationship sex can be directed outward so that the concern is more with the partner than with oneself. The resulting warmth and closeness may be one of the most important sources of contentment, and its absence a cause of great distress. Sexuality can also be used destructively, sometimes as a means of gaining power over the partner, and negative sexual relationships of this sort can damage the quality of life.

Sexuality in later life

We live in a society whose values are largely youth-oriented and in which a powerful emphasis is placed on sex. As a result, there is often an unthinking equation of sex with youth and vigour and a widespread assumption that elderly people are 'past' sexual activity. Indeed, there is even the view that any form of sexual activity on the part of elderly people is intrinsically disgusting. But sexuality is so fundamental in human nature – indeed in all mammalian nature – that it is not going to go away. Sexual interest is as perennial as life itself. Older people, for reasons of discretion, dignity, patience and an awareness of their declining attractiveness, will tacitly conform to this stereotype and will never protest their rights. In this way, the myth of elderly sexlessness is perpetuated.

But the elderly are not sexless. Many older people are more aware of their sexuality than they were when younger. There may, perhaps be less emphasis on the erotic elements and on physical beauty, with more concern for character and achievement. But the preoccupation, nevertheless, is with a member of the opposite sex and the emotions involved may be every bit as strong as those felt by younger people.

Age has other disadvantage particularly its effects on the physical ability to express sexuality. Men worry about their potency and women about their fading looks and it is true that physical sexual power declines gradually with age, especially in men. But the belief that there is an exactly corresponding decline in sexual interest is mistaken. The decline in sexual activity is more often because of loss of opportunity than because of lack of inclination. The belief that the menopause signals the end of a woman's sexual life is another common myth. In fact, the relief from the risk of pregnancy commonly leads to a new and more satisfying phase of the sex life.

Sexual feelings do not disappear just because a person has had a stroke and may be disabled. The need for sexual expression may even be greater after a stroke and this fact cannot be ignored. The aspirations, feelings and desires may be very strongly experienced even if there is no possibility of physical expression, and to ignore or be unaware of this may cause much harm to a relationship. On the other hand, because it is the state of mind that matters, a reduction in the ability to express sexual feeling physicallly may be less important than one might imagine.

In 1974 the Association to Aid the Sexual and Personal Relationships of the Disabled (SPOD) carried out an intensive study of the sexual problems of disabled people. This was the largest research project of its kind ever carried out and the results were as significant as they were sad. Over half of the disabled interviewed had severe sexual problems, damaging to their happiness. And the more severe the disability the worse the difficulties experienced in obtaining sexual satisfaction. Many of these problems arose from defective mental and emotional attitudes towards sex and the disability. And many of the people interviewed were badly in need of advice, help and encouragement.

As in all human endeavour, it is the state of mind and the quality of the motivation which decree the outcome. Enlightenment, determination, courage are needed. There must be open and realistic attitudes to sex and the conviction that, even with disability, a full and gratifying expression of love through sex is possible.

THE EFFECT OF STROKE ON SEXUAL ACTIVITY

There are several reasons why normal sexual expression may be affected by stroke. As we have seen, a stroke is a profoundly alarming and depressing experience which tends to turn people inwards and away from others. This reaction commonly involves a reduction in sexual energy, and severely depressed patients may even lose all interest in sex. The idea of self-image is also important in this context. A person who has suffered loss of physical capacity as a result of a stroke will often have a damaged body image and be unable to believe that he or she is still sexually attractive. If the healthy partner can make the sufferer feel that he or she is still important, accepted and desired as a person, all may be well.

There is a widespread belief that sexual intercourse is actually dangerous to a patient who has had a stroke, in that it may involve a risk of a further attack. The risk is very small and certainly does not justify abstinence if sexual feelings are strong. There have been a few cases, in men, in which a stroke has occurred during intercourse and, as one might imagine, people to whom this has happened are not likely to want to take the risk again. The danger is mainly from the sharp rise in blood pressure during the male orgasm, but the same kind of pressure rise can result from a wide variety of causes, many of them unavoidable. Any strong emotion or sudden physical strain may raise the blood pressure and, since strokes do not recur every time this happens, it follows that the danger is not great. But it is sensible to try to take sex calmly. Men, especially, should avoid over-energetic sexual activity, leaving much of the work to the cooperative partner. The intensity of the orgasm, too, is to some extent under voluntary control.

Older men do not reach orgasm so easily and it is important to dismiss the notion that sex is incomplete or unsatisfactory without an orgasm. This is often merely a matter of pride, related to the significance of retained fertility. If the woman experiences orgasm this may often be a happy point at which to stop. It is deeply satisfying, to most men, to induce an orgasm in the partner.

During stroke, damage may be done to those parts of the brain concerned with sexual responses, but it is important not to make assumptions about this, as there are many other causes of loss of libido, some of which are remediable. Sensory nerve damage, too, can interfere with normal sexual sensation so that much of the physical satisfaction of sex is lost, with severe frustration or waning interest. It is most important for the healthy partner to be aware that skin caressing, on the anaesthetic side, is pointless and may even be emotionally damaging. The partner must concentrate on the feeling side. Actual paralysis need not be such a severe barrier to satisfactory sexual expression as one might think, particularly when the partner is well-motivated, loving and imaginative.

Stroke sometimes causes such a profound change in personality that a partner may feel that he or she is living with a different person – often, although not always, a less pleasant one. This can certainly cause difficulties. It is not uncommon for the personality change to involve a much greater interest in sexual expression than before. This is sometimes directed away from home, and grave inter-personal problems, calling for great strength of character and tolerance, may arise. Medical advice will be warranted in such cases.

The effects of stroke may make the patient much less attractive than before. And, in cases where physical dependence is great, the need for the partner to provide constant bodily attendance may have a negative effect on interest in sex. Much depends on to what extent the patient retains the love, respect and affection of the partner and this, of course, will depend on the degree of mental change. One cannot live indefinitely on memories of past attitudes and, regrettably, it may often be true that the stroke victim has become, in more ways than one, 'a different person'. Such tragedies may have no remedy.

SEXUAL POTENCY AFTER STROKE

Fear of losing sexual pleasure is justified, but it is a mistake for a man, for example, to equate sexual power with masculinity and status as a male. The macho impulse dies hard and is rather primitive. Loss of potency can result from so many causes that it is very difficult, even after full medical investigation, to be sure of the cause. As a general rule, if the bowel and bladder control are retained, then the organic sexual function should be unimpaired. Erection and ejaculation can operate satisfactorily even if the lower part of the spinal cord is completely disconnected from the brain by an injury such as a fractured spine.

However, organic factors other than the effects of the stroke may be operating. For instance, if there is high blood pressure which needs to be treated, the drugs used may cause some loss of potency. Some of the new, more selective, drugs used for high blood pressure are much less liable to have this effect. Many stroke patients are diabetic and this is a fairly common cause of impotence in the male. Other drugs which may cause impotence are alcohol, barbiturates, sedatives such as Valium, drugs used in the treatment of cancer and Parkinsonism, Cimetidine, Lithium and various drugs used for depression and other mental disorders.

Age has an effect on sexual capacity and some degree of loss is entirely normal. Studies have shown that at least a quarter of all men of seventy or over have experienced a substantial loss of capacity, even in the absence of any organic disorder. This usually means an inability to obtain or to sustain a full erection, and this problem may call for more direct and positive genital stimulation than before. But, again, one must be wary of jumping to conclusions, for many such men have been shown to be capable of a full erection during sleep.

The principle cause of impotence following stroke, however, remains the psychological effect of the catastrophe on the victim. In most cases, the remedy is, literally, in the hands of the partner. The loving embrace, the caress, sexually stimulating touching and holding – all potent symbols of caring and need – are the best treatments for psychological impotence. Anxiety must be dispelled, relaxation and freedom of touch encouraged, humour promoted and patience enjoined. Failure must never be made a cause of overt distress.

HEMIPLEGIA AND SEXUAL INTERCOURSE

The physical difficulties of sex after a stroke are a challenge which should be met by free discussion, if necessary with medical advice, and a determination to achieve mutual satisfaction to the fullest possible extent. Full sexual intercourse may be impossible, but that is no reason for assuming that sex is impossible. Men must remember their partners' needs and appreciate that, for most women, sexual interest and desire are hardly affected by age and certainly not by the menopause.

Mutual concern is vital to success. The most powerfully erotic stimulus to one's own sexuality is the sexual excitement of one's partner. Unless the stroke patient is so severely disabled as to be virtually motionless, he or she must remember that his or her own contribution is essential. This is very much a case in which sound investment pays good dividends.

The variety of sexual positions available to the hemiplegic person is, of course, limited. If the disabled person is the man, it will generally be necessary for the woman to take a more active part than she may have done in the past. She may find it necessary to become the dominant partner and may do this both in a physical sense and also by taking the initiative in love-making. This can also add variety and interest.

If the woman is the stroke victim, imaginative and thoughtful amendment in technique may be necessary. Prudery and 'hang-ups' about discussing and changing methods and positions can deny much-needed satisfaction and comfort. The range of positions is far wider than most people imagine even for those suffering a physical handicap. A slavish restriction to the 'missionary position' may be the cause of much unnecessary deprivation. There is no reason, nowadays, except for shyness or inhibition, why anyone should not have access to a great range of information on the subject of sex. Scores of books have been produced and no one need be bashful about purchasing such helpful aids.

Prudish attitudes to masturbation should, if possible, be dispelled as this natural activity is a means of achieving sexual satisfaction for those so disabled as to be incapable of full intercourse. Masturbation, skilfully performed by a partner, can be an eloquent expression of love and regard.

Oral sex may also be important, remembering that respect for the partner's attitudes to this is essential. When oro-genital sex is acceptable to both, it may prove an effective solution to an otherwise insoluble problem.

SEXUAL TECHNIQUE

The whole area of the skin is potentially sexually sensitive and whether or not it becomes so depends largely on the human sensitivity and enlightenment of the partners. Those who hasten to immediate genital contact, or engage in sex fully clothed, are not only omitting an essential stage in the process of arousal but are also denying themselves a great deal of pleasure. Imaginative and patient touching, holding, stroking and caressing can form the basis of greatly heightened sensuality. Experiment, open-mindedness and a willingness to make one's response clear, are necessary. No part of the body should be considered taboo and often it will be found that tactile stimulation of the most unexpected areas may give intense pleasure. Interestingly, those areas most likely to be avoided by the prudish, may be the most productive of pleasure and a sense of intimacy. Unequivocal attention to parts of the body secretly thought to be uninteresting or unattractive to the other, may be very good for the ego and, in turn, for the attitude towards the partner.

But never forget the warning about the importance of the awareness of sensory loss. Remember that the hemi-anaesthetic stroke patient often considers that the unfeeling part of his or her body does not 'belong'. A little absent-mindedness, and your partner might think you are making love to someone else.

Many disabled men who have suffered reduced libido require stimulation to be applied with both sensitivity and continuity. It may be difficult for the man to convey this to his partner, for any attempt on his part to guide her may have a negative effect. Discussion is essential. Skin stimulation, when effective, will produce at least some degree of erection and this must be cherished and promoted by a progress to direct, tactile stimulation of the penis. All too often, a promising erection may be lost. Often it will be necessary for the woman to sustain the penile stimulation right up to the point of insertion and, even then, any fumbling or delay may be fatal. The method of penile stimulation must also be skilful and acceptable to the man. There is no substitute for frank discussion and demonstration.

Inadequate erection is common, but this need not prevent rewarding sex. The strongest stimulus to erection is the feeling of penetration. One way or another this should be achieved – even by limp 'stuffing'! Vaginal lubrication is important and is in itself strongly stimulating to the man. If nature needs some help, try K-Y gel. This has become so popular for this purpose that the manufacturers feel obliged to print on the tube, 'This is NOT a contraceptive'! Every pharmacist sells it and it is very safe.

Sexual positioning is dealt with comprehensively in other books, but imagination is cheaper. The principles are that nothing is unnatural except that which causes pain or distress and that variety is the spice of loving. Within the limits imposed by disability, the greater the variety the better.

GETTING FURTHER HELP

It is surprising how much can often be done for stroke patients with sexual problems if the barrier of shyness or embarrassment can be overcome and advice sought. This is most easily achieved by applying to an organisation specifically concerned to deal with these problems in a matter-of-fact manner. Such an organisation is the Association to Aid the Sexual and Personal Relationships of the Disabled (SPOD), 186 Camden Road, London N7 0BJ. SPOD has been running since 1972 and has considerable experience in handling problems of this kind. Since carrying out the major survey on the sexual problems of the disabled, the Association has successfully supplied advice through a large number of counsellors throughout the country. Anyone needing such advice should contact SPOD who will probably be able to put them in touch with one of their people.

In addition to this service, SPOD supply a series of advisory leaflets on the sexual problems of the disabled. These include pamphlets on the general subject of physical disability and sex; on positions for sexual intercourse for disabled people; on aids to sex for the handicapped; on sex for the severely disabled and on advice for those looking after a physically handicapped person.

Another very helpful organisation is The National Marriage Guidance Council, Little Church Street, Rugby CV21 3AP, which offers counselling to any person with marital or sexual problems and runs Sexual Dysfunction clinics. There are more than 500 counselling centres throughout the country with nearly 2000 counsellors, some with special knowledge of the sexual problems of disabled people. Those not living in Britain should make enquiries about similar organisations in their own countries. Help will always be available to those willing to ask for it.

In the USA, the following organisations are concerned with the sexual problems of the disabled, as well as with marriage guidance:

The Alan Guttmacher Institute,
360 Park Avenue South,
New York, NY 10010
Tel 212-685-5858

Sex Information and Educational Council of the United States,
Suite 801, 80 Fifth Avenue,
New York, NY 10011
Tel 212-929-2300

Sister Kenny Institute,
Abbott-Northwestern Hospital,
2727 Chicago Avenue,
Minneapolis, MN 55407
Tel 612-874-4175

8 Technology Can Help

Technology can help stroke patients in a number of different ways and many ideas involve very low technology indeed. It can help in rehabilitation, in compensating for various forms of physical disability, in providing entertainment not otherwise available and, above all, it can help in communication. But first, a mention of one or two very useful gadgets which can make life a great deal easier for those who have to manage with one hand.

KITCHEN AIDS FOR THE HEMIPLEGIC

There has been a lot of progress in the design of special implements for the one-handed but many useful gadgets, not designed with them in mind, are available in hardware stores. It is surprising how easily some domestic implements can be adapted to hemiplegic use. There is, for instance, a very handy wall-mounted gadget for taking off screw caps. This uses a strong, adjustable composition plastic strap which can be tightened round almost any size of screw cap. It is fixed to the device at one end and free at the other. Once the strap is applied, the bottle or jar may be turned with one hand. The same gadget can be used for other holding purposes.

Small vices are available which can be attached to the edge of a table and which have holding clamps adjustable to any position. They are popular with people doing fine work and are sold by firms dealing in electronic parts for constructors. Other useful aids are wall-mounted can openers, some of them electrically operated; electric carving knives; and electric irons which have no cord to get in the way, but which pick up current and boost the heat each time they are laid down on the special stand. Many such devices designed for the able-bodied are of special value to the disabled. Further ideas are given in Chapter 11, especially in the section on gardening.

An immense amount of thought and care has gone into developing devices specially designed for the one-handed and all kinds of ideas have been developed. Before considering these in detail, some further useful kitchen aids should be mentioned.

Many simple devices to hold things like potatoes and apples, for preparation, are possible. For instance, if a few clean two-inch nails are driven through a board, the fruit or vegetable can be stuck on the spikes and cut one-handed. The same board may have two short pieces of beading to form a raised edge at one corner so that slices of bread can be secured for margarining (people who have had strokes don't eat butter). Such boards are even more useful if fitted with rubber sucker feet to prevent them from moving. Special knives are available for the one-handed, working on the rocking rather than the sawing principle, and these may also be helpful while eating. Plate guards can be clipped on to plates to prevent food from being pushed off. Non-slip mats, pan holders, even suction cups can be very helpful to stabilise objects in the kitchen so that they can be used one-handed.

There is an ingenious egg-cup with which the one-handed can lift an egg out of the boiling water and secure it firmly for one-handed eating. Some of these egg-cups have a rubber sucker base by which they can be firmly held on a smooth surface. There are saucepans with magnetic feet to hold them firm while the contents are being stirred; levers for turning taps, keys, latches, etc; electric plugs with handles on the back which make them much easier to insert and remove – no end of helpful gadgets.

Such aids can prevent disabled people from developing a sense of helplessness or uselessness. It is critical to contentment and peace of mind to be able to contribute usefully in the home and be spared the sense of being a burden to others.

HELP IN THE SITTING ROOM

People whose movements are restricted are very dependent on the telephone for maintaining essential contact with relatives and friends. A very useful device in this context is the telephone shoulder rest into which the receiver can be clipped so that the hand is freed. The need to hold the receiver can be dispensed with altogether by using an instrument incorporating an amplifier and a loud-speaker so that one can talk and listen some distance from the phone. Advantage can also be taken of the recent improvement in telephone design. Press-button 'dialling', memory systems which store twenty or more commonly used numbers, automatic SOS calling by pressing one button, and facilities which will automatically recall an unobtainable number – all these advantages are now commonplace and can be obtained quite cheaply.

New telephones can simply be plugged in, in place of the old.

For those with artistic inclinations it is even possible to make some use of the paralysed arm. The forearm is laid in a light plastic 'gutter' support which has four ball-bearing runners on its under side. The arm is secured with two Velcro bands and the wrist is tilted back a little into the proper anti-spasm position. But the real point of the gadget is that it has a holder at the level of the fingertips for a pencil or a paintbrush or some other tool. Because the gutter can move freely over any smooth surface, those hemiplegics who retain shoulder movement – and this is very common – can, albeit with difficulty, write or paint or perform other useful tasks with the weak arm, even if the hand is entirely useless.

This is the modern version of a system of suspension of the arm on strings and pulleys and is simple and cheap. Some people prefer to have the support for the weak arm suspended on balanced cords, but this requires some sort of overhead structure and limits mobility. Frames on castors can be obtained which can be placed close behind the chair. From these are suspended the supporting cords and either springs or counterpoise weights may be used to cancel the effects of gravity on the paralysed arm. Activities made possible by devices of this sort should always be encouraged.

Many patients have difficulty in getting out of comfortable armchairs, and chairs with mechanisms for raising the sitter into an almost vertical position are invaluable. They may be electrically operated or use a simple tilting seat principle. The Rolls Royce versions of these chairs also enable the person to recline into a lying position and may even have electrically operated leg rests. There are comfortable chairs with 'gliders' – efficient castors which make it easy for them to be pushed about the room even under the full weight of the stroke patient. And, for those who wish to use a tray across the knees, there is an ingenious 'bean bag' table of which the supporting part moulds itself to the knees and thighs while the upper, formica covered surface can easily be set horizontally or at a tilt, as required.

HELP IN THE BATHROOM

Hand-grips can be of enormous value throughout the home. Carefully placed, and firmly attached with rawlplugs, suitable metal grips provide a cheap and wonderfully helpful aid. They are easily secured to almost any surface and they should especially be considered in the toilet and bathroom where they might make the difference between independence and humiliating reliance on others. The problems of the hemiplegic person in the bathroom are important. Getting into and out of the bath may pose so many problems that it is often better to resort to a secure bathboard set across the width, on which to sit while washing. I emphasise 'secure'. Such boards should be designed so that they can neither slip into the bath nor turn sideways. Used in conjunction with a hand-held shower with rubber attachments for the bath taps, the daily all-over wash becomes a practical possibility with a gain in morale. Lost soap can be a problem and 'soap on a rope' is a good idea. Back-scrubbing is difficult even for someone without hemiplegia, and a long-handled brush is useful. A non-slip bath mat is essential.

For the affluent, hoists and bath lifters are available by means of which the hemiplegic person can be gently lowered into the water and, when finished, hoisted out again.

Shaving with the left hand can be difficult, but skill will come with practice. Men and women who are accustomed to razors may find it an advantage to switch to electric shavers which can easily be used with the unaccustomed hand.

Toilet privacy is, of course, greatly valued, and hemiplegic patients unable to attend to themselves will bless the designers of the automatic WC which can flush-wash the nether regions with warm water and then apply a blow of hot air to dry the bottom – a sort of super-bidet. There are various other appliances to facilitate cleansing. There are even gadgets which enable menstruating women who cannot insert tampons to do so. Commodes are very convenient for those who cannot safely go far from the bed. These come in a bewildering variety of designs and some incorporate a chemical system to sterilise and deodorise the contents after use.

AIDS TO GETTING ABOUT

Wheelchairs, leg braces, crutches, walking frames, quadripods and ordinary walking sticks can be of considerable value to those who cannot manage without them, but it is a great mistake to adopt these aids prematurely while there is still the possibility of managing without. But there will be many who have reached the limit of their improvement, and aids to mobility can be invaluable for them. Some important facts about these aids may be helpful.

WHEELCHAIRS

These come in all degrees of sophistication and price. Many can be folded to fit into a small space such as a car boot or the limited space of a small invalid vehicle. Modern electronic control of battery power and developments in battery technology have greatly improved the design of self-powered wheelchairs so that steering and speed can even be controlled by moving a small lever with one finger. The battery can be charged at night simply by plugging into the mains, but a spare should be kept in case of failure. Powered wheelchairs use smaller wheels than self-propelled chairs and their tires are usually thicker and give a very soft ride. They come in three main types:

● Those intended for indoor use which require smooth surfaces to run on and cannot negotiate even slightly raised obstructions.
● Those for general purpose outdoor use, capable of travelling across rough ground and mounting kerbs. Many of these chairs are too wide and long to be used conveniently indoors.
● An intermediate design capable of good indoor performance, but limited in difficult outdoor conditions.

With self-propelled chairs it is important to ensure that the tyres are always properly inflated and this is most conveniently done with a small mains-operated pump. If the tyres are allowed to go soft, the chair will require much more force to move it and the brakes may not work. Insecure brakes can be dangerous especially when the owner is getting in or out of the chair.

AIDS TO WALKING

Walking frames are made of very light alloy but are amply strong enough to bear the whole weight of the patient. Although they give excellent support they do not allow for more than very slow progress and great patience is needed. Walking frames tend to get in the way of the feet, and do not encourage normal walking. If weight can be taken on the arm on the affected side, elbow crutches should be substituted as soon as possible.

Elbow crutches can be very useful, but should also be looked on as a transitional aid to mobility. They can be used in a number of ways. People who are shaky and insecure should start with 'four point' walking. The four points are the two feet and the two crutch tips and this gives high stability. Only one foot, or one crutch moves at a time and the sequence of forward movement, starting with the two crutch tips well ahead of the feet, is: right foot, left foot, right crutch, left crutch.

From this secure but slow sequence the patient can graduate to 'three point' walking in which the weight is taken on the sound leg while both crutches are moved forward together. The weight is then taken on the crutches while the affected foot is allowed to swing forward. If the foot on the hemiplegic side cannot take weight at all, there is another form of 'three point' walking. Here the two crutches go forward together and the weight is taken on both while both legs swing through. In 'two point' walking, the right foot and the left crutch move forward together, then the left foot and the right crutch together.

Crutches can cause problems on the stairs and great care is needed to place the crutch tip well back from the edge of the tread. A crutch slipping off a tread can lead to a serious accident. Placing the crutch tip well back tends to make one lean forward and this is safe when going upstairs, but should be avoided when coming down. It is best to make full use of the banister rail, for support, and it will be easier when this is on the weak side so that one crutch can be used on the strong side with the second crutch tucked under the arm. If the banister rail is on the strong side when coming downstairs, it may be better to turn and come down backwards so as to have the benefit of the fullest support. If children are about, watch out for toys or other small objects left on the stair treads and be especially careful if the nap of the carpet tends to catch the tip of the crutch.

Quadripod walking sticks are especially useful if there is difficulty with balance. The four little feet give a stable support on which one can lean and, once the balance is sure, the stick can be swung forward for walking. Some similar models are made with only three feet, but these are not to be recommended as they are much less stable. The quadripod stick is helpful as a transitional device between crutches and the ordinary walking stick, but, again, the area of the base, while good for balance, can obstruct foot movement.

Of all aids to mobility, the ordinary walking stick is certainly the most useful, but this, too, should be discarded as soon as one can manage without. It is important that the walking stick should be the correct length so that the posture may be as upright as possible, with neither forward nor sideways lean. The length should allow a slight bend at the elbow. Some light alloy walking sticks are adjustable, but these must be non-collapsible. A firm rubber tip is desirable as is a comfortable grip.

The best way for a hemiplegic person to use a walking stick is to hold it in the hand on the strong side and to follow the natural swing of the arm so that the stick is forward as the weak foot comes to the ground and the weight of the body can be shared between the stick and the weak leg. To begin with, most of the weight will tend to be taken on the stick, but one should always try to share the weight so that the weak leg is exercised and heavy limping avoided. If the arm on the weak side is strong enough to take the strain, an alternative way is to use the stick as a sort of splint for the weak leg, holding it close to and parallel with the weak leg so that the two come to the ground together. In this way, the stick supports the weak leg.

A lot of emphasis has been put on the importance of positioning to avoid spasm and the resulting abnormal positions of the limbs. But in spite of the best of intentions, many people will end up with foot drop and inversion so that the toes will tend to catch on the ground making natural walking very difficult. For these, some form of foot support may be essential. Various supports are available and it is seldom necessary to resort to the clumsy and ugly external metal braces formerly used. Special footwear may be used to prevent ankle extension, or light plastic splints may be worn inside normal shoes. If calipers are worn to control foot drop, they must be carefully fitted and properly adjusted to the individual. Chafing of the longitudinal iron pieces against the leg must not be permitted as this may cause great discomfort or even, if there is sensory loss, ulceration of the skin.

HIGH TECHNOLOGY AIDS TO COMMUNICATION

The plight of the stroke victim in full possession of mental powers, but unable to speak, is a dire one and any device allowing communication will be of great value. Early attempts to aid communication were painfully slow and cumbersome, most of them involving some sort of letter board or word list on which the desired letter or word could be indicated by pointing. This was dreadfully slow and frustrating. Today's communication aids are becoming ever more sophisticated and readily available. A major breakthrough occurred with the development of cheap speech synthesisers and these now form the basis of most modern communication systems for the speechless.

Speech synthesisers have become possible as a result of the staggering increase in the amount of data which can be stored in the electronic chips called 'read only memories' (ROMs). ROMs programmed with short word lists are now so cheap that they are commonly found in toys. These tiny chips can be used in two different ways. Either they can be stored with data corresponding to complete words, or stored with smaller packets of data corresponding to all the basic sounds (phonemes) from which words are made up. In the first case, the chip will have a vocabulary limited to the number of words which can be accommodated – perhaps one or two hundred. In the system using stored phonemes there is no limit to the number of words which can be produced, but, of course, the system must provide a means of deciding which phonemes are needed and then some way of stringing them together to make intelligible words.

In both cases the synthesiser employs a microprocessor to organise the way in which the required addresses in the ROM, in which the words or phonemes are stored, are looked up and the contents retrieved. Clearly the system storing complete words is much simpler, and a communicator might consist simply of a word board, on which the required word can be indicated by touch or other means, the ROM, the microprocessor, a way of converting the digital data from the ROM into analogue signals, a low-power amplifier and a small loudspeaker. But such a system has limited use as only the words built in are available. The phoneme system, on the other hand, really needs a computer with a fair amount of software to run it, and the input must be in a form which the person using the system is capable of operating. In experimental speech synthesis systems this is usually a standard keyboard and this is not really practical for a stroke-disabled person. If, as is common when there is speech loss, the right hand is paralysed, input will be much too slow and it will not be possible to produce synthesised speech quickly enough.

A compromise between the two systems is possible. Using the phoneme system, the operator can, at leisure, put together desired words, phrases or even complete sentences, and then give each of these a code consisting of one or two letters. A two-letter code will cover seven hundred words, phrases or sentences, and each can be called up by pressing only two keys. This requires a good memory. In chapter 11 is an account of further advances which make it possible for a person who can only operate a single two-way switch to use a standard computer keyboard.

A phrase or sentence in synthesised speech can sound quite natural – heard once. But as travellers on the subway or underground will know, it is the precise repetition of the same sequence of sounds, strung together in exactly the same way, which is unnatural. This aspect is being studied by electronic and acoustic engineers and, although it is perhaps too much to expect that the tones should convey appropriate emotion, at least some random variety in voice quality will be achieved. An important advance has been made by researchers at the Institute for Perception Research in Eindhoven, Holland who have worked out a method of breaking down speech into smaller units than phonemes. These are called 'diphones' and they give much more subtle control over speech synthesis than does the use of phonemes. Diphones flow together to give natural-sounding speech and about two thousand diphones can represent almost any spoken language. As with pictures, the smaller the elements making up the whole, the greater the detail and realism, and so it is with diphones. Patients may look forward confidently to ever more natural synthesised speech, and aphasic people, using such devices are likely to produce voices of better quality than before the stroke!

MICROS FOR PERSONAL COMMUNICATION

A different, and in some ways more versatile, approach to communication is by way of the monitor screen. Microcomputers are now so cheap that this has become a reasonable and economical proposition for people of limited means. In many cases, a printer will not be required and that will almost halve the cost. There are many ways in which the microcomputer revolution has improved life for people disabled by stroke. More of these are dealt with in Chapter 11, but here we are concerned only with the important question of communication. Graham Goodge's case shows how important this is.

HOW GRAHAM'S LIFE WAS CHANGED

Graham had been unlucky at school. He was intelligent enough but didn't seem to get on too well with his teachers and, as a result, felt little encouragement to work. He spent a lot of time in class day-dreaming. He was an imaginative boy but paid very little attention to his studies and had left school, soon after the war, with three rather poor 'O' level passes. He had tried various jobs such as working in an insurance office and a house agent's business – but hadn't settled in any of them. He had even tried to sell household brushes from door to door. For a while he had a reasonably successful business repairing radio and television sets but the arrival of the cheap transistor radio knocked the bottom out of the repair business and Graham was unable to compete with the TV rental schemes.

Things went from bad to worse, and for long periods he was on the dole, living a miserable and seemingly pointless bachelor existence with few friends and very little happiness. Finally, well into his fifties and deeply depressed, he tried to gas himself. But even in this he was unsuccessful. A neighbour smelt the escaping gas, kicked in the flimsy door to his apartment and dragged his unconscious body outside. When Graham came round it was to the realisation that his suicide attempt had precipitated a stroke and that he was paralysed down his right side. Although his mental processes were unimpaired, he had completely lost the power of speech.

In the hospital he met a middle-aged widow, an attractive and lively part-time nurse, and, largely through her efforts, he regained the power of walking and they became friends. Some quality of resignation and helplessness in him appealed to her. Within a few weeks Muriel decided to give up nursing and devote herself to him and they were married. For the first time in his life, Graham found that he had a motive for succeeding, but now he felt that there was nothing he could do about it. Above all, he wanted to communicate with her. He had so much to express, so much love and appreciation for her kindness and support, that it was torture to remain silent, able to express his thoughts only by scrawling awkwardly, with his left hand.

Graham had kept up his interest in electronics and, one day, when he was standing in a shop with Muriel his attention was caught by a home computer display. Idly, he touched a few keys and when Muriel felt a gentle nudge and turned, she saw the words 'I love you, darling.' On the screen. Then, with almost frantic haste, Graham was tapping out a message to her which he had been trying vainly to get across all morning.

The point was not lost on Muriel and she insisted on buying him the computer. It was the beginning of a revolution for Graham. Within a week he had set up his 'coms station' by his armchair and had run a cable under the carpet to a second monitor screen by Muriel's chair. A tactfully quiet bleep – made to sound on Muriel's monitor by pressing one of the control keys – was the signal to attract her attention to the screen, and Graham would usually have the message already on display before sounding it. Muriel would turn, glance at the screen and answer in a manner as natural as if he had spoken to her audibly.

Soon he had mastered the word processing program and was becoming a skilled and rapid, left-hand typist. With this new ease of communication, his confidence and assurance grew and he began to study programming. His first major development was a means of speeding up, even further, the rate of communication with his wife. In a matter of days he had written a basic program which established a large glossary of common phrases in the computer's memory, each one of which could be recalled by a two-letter code and displayed on the monitor screens. So now, his conversations with Muriel were able to proceed at a rate not far short of slow speech.

Muriel had suggested that Graham should join the Chest, Heart and Stroke Association (see Chapter 10) and it occurred to him that his experience might be of interest to other stroke patients, so he started typing a short article for the CHSA newspaper, pointing out the value of the microcomputer as an aid to communication. To his satisfaction, although he had produced the article on a very cheap dot-matrix printer, it was accepted for publication and this encouraged him to consider the possibility of further writing. Several other computer programs now followed and Muriel began to be interested, so he started to explain Basic to her.

The need for economy and clarity in his explanations proved to be a good discipline and, one day, Muriel said, 'I hope you've been saving these explanations.'

'Why?' he asked, on the monitor.

'They're very good. Seems a pity I'm the only one reading them . . .'

Thus was Graham Goodge launched on his one-handed career as a writer on microcomputers. It was the height of the home computer boom and publishers could not get enough material to satisfy the enormous public demand for books on the subject. Graham sold two manuscripts and with the advances was able to upgrade his 'coms station' and buy a good daisy wheel printer. He was now proud of the quality of his manuscripts and further sales soon justified the cost of a photocopier. Muriel was spending more and more of her time helping him. At one stage she considered learning to type but, knowing how much it meant to Graham to be producing his own manuscripts, said nothing.

'If I could use right hand for shift key,' typed Graham, 'Would be lot faster.'

'Well, why don't you?'

'Can't.'

Muriel had seen stroke patients in the rehabilitation department of her hospital sitting under a kind of frame from which were suspended balanced cords to support the paralysed arm, and she suggested something of the sort to Graham.

'If you're only going to use it for the shift key, that should be easy enough.'

'OK' typed Graham.

The outcome exceeded both their expectations and Graham found that, with his right hand supported in a suspended gutter and the fingers carefully positioned, he was able, by dipping his right shoulder, to get his hand so placed that he was able to use his right thumb for the space bar and the index finger for the shift key. Gradually, as his skill increased, he used his right hand more and more. Although it never acquired the speed and accuracy of his left hand, the use of two hands soon had him typing at an almost professional rate.

Graham had found his vocation and never looked back. With Muriel's support and research assistance he later became a successful professional writer of non-fiction with a dozen books and hundreds of magazine articles to his credit.

'No sense of proportion,' said Muriel with a hint of tears in her eyes, as she opened a letter from one of Graham's publishers offering a contract for a new book. 'Making a virtue of necessity isn't enough for you. Oh no! Triumph out of bloody adversity's more your style!'

'Language!' typed Graham, smiling lop-sidedly.

COMPUTERS AND THE FUTURE

Word processing is not the only use of a microcomputer. Indeed, there seems to be no limit to the versatility and applications of these remarkable devices. The microprocessor – the central controlling chip at the heart of the computer – is now so cheap that it is used in all sorts of gadgets and machines. Microprocessors now run automatic washing machines, sewing machines, tape recorders, central heating systems, toys – no end of devices – very much more efficiently, and much more cheaply than was ever possible before.

It is a simple task for a microprocessor to receive information from a dozen different sources – some of it contradictory – weigh up the significance of it in accordance with criteria laid down by the designer and produce in 'real time' (that is, while everything is actually happening) a response which has taken everything into account. Suppose, for example, a powered wheel-chair designer wanted to enable the driver to control speed, steering and braking with a tiny, finger-operated lever; and suppose he wanted to avoid the motor slowing down too much when the chair went up a slope, but not run ahead too quickly when going downhill; and suppose he wanted to prevent the operator from putting the chair into reverse while going forward, or try to move off while the brakes were on; and to give speech-synthesised warning when anything was done wrong. A microprocessor would coordinate all these requirements and do the job standing on its head – and go on doing it for years with complete reliability.

There is enormous scope for the use of microprocessors in aids to people who have had strokes and the applications are limited only by the ingenuity and motivation of the engineer. We can confidently expect wonders in the not too distant future.

9 Other People Have Rights, Too

THE ROLE OF THE FAMILY_____

Doctors are busy people and have their hands full just coping with their acutely ill patients. Of course they are aware of the difficulties experienced by the families of stroke patients, but it is hard to see how they are going to be able to find time to do anything about it. Once a stroke patient is out of danger, the busy hospital doctor can afford to spend very little time with that patient. New patients are constantly coming in and other lives have to be saved. So the job of attending to the new stroke victim has to fall to some member of the family. And, regrettably, however devoted the younger members of the family may be, they will usually have career or marital responsibilities, and it will be unrealistic in most cases to expect them to accept a major caring role.

Sometimes, a daughter or daughter-in-law will accept this task – perhaps at the cost of her career or even the sacrifice of a marriage. But in the great majority of cases, the job is left to the closest one – usually the spouse – on whom falls the responsibility of providing the vital physical attention, comfort and moral support necessary for recovery or even survival. This chapter is dedicated to those who find themselves in this situation.

Like it or not, the carer is stuck with a major task – a task which may alter the whole way of life and, perhaps seriously damage its quality. Because stroke is a condition mainly affecting the elderly, the probability is that both patient and carer are well past their physical prime. Add to that the distress, anxiety and loss of amenity and perhaps income, and the need to take on many tasks formerly the responsibility of the patient, and it is apparent that the carer's burden is a heavy one. No one should be expected to carry this major responsibility without help or advice.

The carer is likely to have had very little preparation for the patient's release from hospital and may have been told hardly anything about the business of looking after an invalid. The District Nurse in Britain, or the Home Care Nurse in the USA, is usually a great help but she is busy too and really hasn't enough time to pass on all that should be known. In addition, the carer is likely to be feeling tired, lonely and greatly in need of a bit of assistance.

HOW MUCH SHOULD THE CARER ENDURE?____

Few carers enjoy any real compensation for the heavy burden imposed on them and many, understandably, feel resentful. But few are willing to express the full degree of resentment felt and this is sometimes a pity as the repression of such very natural and reasonable feelings can make them worse. Of course, the expression of such feelings to the person whose misfortune has caused them would be indefensible, but the honest acceptance of them, and the expression of them to some other understanding person, can be therapeutic. Stroke clubs (see below) can offer an opportunity for the expression of such feelings and it will often be a great relief to find that other people, especially those one respects, have the same kind of feelings.

One person's confession will tend to lead others to admit similar reactions. At one 'stroke relatives' meeting the wife of a stroke victim admitted that she had come to hate her husband because of the severely damaging effect his illness had had on her life. This led another to admit that she had come to believe that it would have been better if her husband had died because she could not bear the life – so terribly damaged by his disability – that they were now leading. Such feelings are natural, logical and widely held and should not cause guilt.

Many heavily burdened carers have asked themselves the question 'How much should I have to take?' The following story may help to answer this question.

The McLeods were a devoted couple who had had a good life together. Ups and downs, of course, like anyone else, but supportive and caring and on the whole very happy. David McLeod was a Naval architect and had spent most of his working life in Admiralty dockyards and his wife Constance had borne with patience and good humour the many moves from Rosyth to Malta and from Gibraltar to Hong Kong. But she had always looked forward to the day when they could finally settle down in Scotland in a little bungalow of their own and make a proper home.

At last, David retired on pension and they bought a house in Tayport – rather larger than Constance would have chosen, but they could afford it and David had always been rather inclined to ostentation. David was building a patio extension and Constance went out with a cup of coffee to find him lying on a heap of wet cement, breathing noisily and with his face all lop-sided and twisted.

The Consultant at Dundee Royal Infirmary spoke to her gravely. 'Aye, well, it's a pretty massive stroke, I'm afraid. He's had a big cerebral haemorrhage, and ye must prepare yourself for the worse.'

'You think he's going to die, then?' asked Constance, desperately trying to control herself.

'Yes I do. I'm afraid there's very little hope for him.'

But the Consultant was wrong and David did not die. After two or three days on the critical list, he recovered consciousness and, although he was unable to speak, Constance was overjoyed to discover that he could recognise her and could communicate in writing, using his left hand. At first, David's progress was rapid and, within a week he had recovered, not only the power of speech, but also nearly normal strength on his right side. His character, however, seemed to have changed and, from being a positive-minded, dominant man he had become weakly and apparently wholly lacking in motivation. A month after his admission, David was discharged from hospital and Constance gladly welcomed him back to their home overlooking the broad reach of the river Tay.

Constance was fit and healthy but she was a small woman and David's sixteen stones of passive weight presented problems. Had he been his usual self, he would have relished the problem and probably come up with a bright idea for some sort of hoist. But Constance was not getting any cooperation and he just lay there looking at her resentfully as if the whole thing were her fault. It was a difficult effort even to turn him over in bed, but this had to be done frequently because, apart from the question of bed-sores, David was doubly incontinent and soiled the bedlinen several times a day.

Although he could speak, his remarks were confined to self-pitying complaints. Soon after returning home he established the habit of crying out for Constance in a high-pitched voice whenever he had the slightest inclination. Often there seemed to be no reason for this but Constance could not bring herself to ignore him and always went to him. He was especially prone to call her during the night – Constance had had to retire to the guest bedroom because of his incontinence and his restlessness – and she soon reached near-exhaustion from lack of sleep.

Constance was a person of great strength of character and was determined to do her duty. She was an optimist and expected every day that some improvement would occur so that she might see some possibility of an end to her perpetual and thankless task. But the weeks passed and, in spite of her every effort and the regular exhortations of the District Nurse, David could never be persuaded to cooperate in anything and refused even to allow her to try to get him out of bed.

Constance knew that such behaviour was quite out of character and generously attributed it, not to his selfish stubbornness, but to the effects of the brain damage. Even so, it was very difficult for her not to respond as if he were fully responsible and she constantly had to repress an impulse to angry protest.

'There's no actual physical reason why he should not get out of bed,' the District Nurse told her, 'He has full muscle power on both sides and could walk fine if he wanted. This lying in bed is dangerous and it would be very good for him if he would get up.'

'Good for me, too,' thought Constance a little bitterly.

For several weeks Constance conscientiously carried out her task of keeping David clean, seeing that he moved his limbs frequently, and turning him many times a day. Then the visits of the District Nurse became less regular and finally stopped and Constance felt that she had been abandoned. Unhappily, David had shown little improvement and continued to behave in a childish and inconsiderate manner, demanding her constant attention and showing no sign of appreciation for what she was doing for him. In an attempt to reduce the work caused by his incontinence, she had obtained special, tight-fitting incontinence garments for him, but unless she watched him closely he would always try to pull them off.

Gradually, Constance's anger grew – anger against the fate that had brought her this lonely, thankless drudgery instead of the serene peace she had expected in her declining years; anger against the indifference of her few friends, none of whom apparently had any idea of the dreadful life she was leading; anger against David's relatives who had steadfastly refused to help; and, in the end, and in spite of the promptings of her better nature, anger against David himself. Although tied to him by a deep sense of duty, and constantly in his company, she was profoundly lonely for he offered her no companionship – nothing but endless unpleasant labour and regularly disturbed sleep.

Finally, one day, when, within half an hour of stripping his bed and putting everything in the wash, she went in to find that David had again soiled voluminously, Constance's restraint broke.

'You're doing it on purpose,' she stormed out at the grinning man in the bed, 'I don't believe you're half as bad as you pretend to be. You can just damn well lie in it!'

Half an hour later, she relented and went back, washed him and changed his bed linen, but by now she had come to a decision.

'The doctor says you are able to get up and should get up.'

'Can't,' said David.

'I have rights, too, you know,' said Constance, 'And this is when I start exercising them.'

With sudden resolution she flung back the duvet. 'Roll over to the side of the bed!' she ordered.

'Can't.'

Constance went to the far side of the bed and with a strength she did not know she possessed, heaved up the edge of the mattress so that David half rolled, half slid across to the edge. At that point she hardly cared whether he fell out of bed or not.

'What're you doing?' he asked querulously.

Constance compressed her lips, took hold of his ankles and swung his legs over the side of the bed.'

'You'll do me an injury.' protested David weakly.

'Nonsense!' With a supreme effort, Constance forced him into a sitting position and stood back, leaving him to balance or fall over as he chose. David chose to balance and sat, precariously with his hands on the edge of the bed.

'Now get up on your feet!'

'No way!' I'll never stand up again. Ye don't seem t'understand that I've had a stroke.'

'From which you've made an almost complete recovery,' said Constance.

'I can't stand! I'm paralysed!'

'Nonsense! Get up!'

David tried to fall back on the bed, but Constance grabbed his hands and pulled so that he fell forward on to his knees.

'Now look what you've done!' he cried.

Something inspired Constance to stand back and leave him. 'You couldn't stay like that if you were paralysed.' she said firmly, 'You'd better get up on your feet.' She went over to the window and turned her back on him.

'What's got into you?' asked David, 'Don't you love me any more?'

'No I don't!' said Constance, 'You're not the man you were. And I'm fed up with your selfishness. You'd better start fending for yourself because I'm not going to be your skivvy any more.'

David began to walk towards her on his knees and when she heard the sound she turned, went across to him and, with a feeling close to desperation, put her arms round his waist and dragged him up on to his feet. When she let go of him, he stood swaying for a moment. Constance looked at his face and watched the slowly dawning expression of surprise mixed with shame. It was the first time for months that she had had evidence of any concern beyond the purely selfish and it was, for her, a moment of deep joy. She went to him and took him in her arms.

David's real recovery dated from that critical moment, and within a few weeks he was back working on the patio and giving a hand with the housework.

It should not be inferred from this story that many stroke patients are malingering. But it is important to grasp that the majority are likely, if not pushed quite hard, to do much less for themselves than they are capable of. There are many reasons for this, some psychological and related to the sense of resentment suffered by most stroke victims ('Why should this happen to me?'), and some the result of organic brain damage affecting the will to action. It is very bad for patients to fall into a kind of hopeless lethargy. There is no doubt at all that the end result may be radically different if proper pressure is applied to stroke patients to make them TRY.

The kind of life the carer enjoys (or suffers) depends very much on the patient's needs. Regrettably, only too often, the whole purpose of a carer's life centres around concern for the patient. Whatever the circumstances, however, a carer is entitled to a private life and some measure of private satisfaction.

The relationship of the carer to the patient is often complex. On the one hand there is dependence and need and, on the other, constant giving. But dependence does not always promote the gratitude one might reasonably expect. Sometimes it breeds resentment, particularly in people formerly self-reliant and capable. Such resentment is difficult to take and may lead to resentment in the carer. So the more the stroke patient can achieve alone, the better the relationship.

It is also very important for the carer to have some independence in another sense. At least some time – ideally one day a week – must, at all costs, be spent away from the patient. This is not as heartless as it sounds. Much experience has shown that an intolerable situation can be made bearable if there is a regular break to give relief. This is something a carer is entitled to expect and demand, but how it is achieved is another matter. Local authorities run day care centres, minders can be found – paid or volunteer; it may even be possible to organise a minder rota through a stroke club or stroke relatives club. Temporarily exchanging responsibility for one person for responsibility for another may not seem much of a deal. But change can add variety and interest and may be almost as good as a rest.

It may be possible to get some time off by moving one stroke patient temporarily to the house of another so that one carer can attend to two patients. Such arrangements are really only feasible for members of a friendly stroke club. Members of these clubs have a common purpose in improving the quality of life, both for the victims and the carers, and will always consider such suggestions positively.

PRIVACY

This is another difficult question likely to lead to soul-searching because of the inevitable conflict of rights and duties. Should the carer, for instance, insist on having his or her own bedroom? Human company and sex may be very important to both but to one forced to be in the presence of a demanding patient throughout most of the day, there may be a strong need for night-time privacy. Day-time privacy, too, can be important for mental comfort, and having somewhere to retire to, if only for an hour or so at a time, can recharge emotional batteries. This will not usually be a problem if the patient remains in bed during the day, but if the patient spends all day in the sitting room, it may be necessary to explain, kindly but firmly, that one needs to be alone from time to time.

Gardening can be an ideal way of combining privacy with an absorbing and refreshing interest and offers a diplomatic means of getting away for a time. Gardens must not be allowed to fall into neglect, so regular attention is needed.

THE PATIENT MAY DIE

One must recognise that the mortality rate, in people who have had strokes, is quite high and the possibility of death within the foreseeable future, must always be considered. The carer must think of the future and it is important not to put all concern into the one activity of caring, to the exclusion of all possible future interests. An absorbing occupation is essential for happiness, and it is difficult for the busy carer to pursue such occupation. Many try to achieve satisfaction in caring. But it is dangerous to arrange one's life wholly around an occupation which might suddenly be withdrawn.

It is not heartless to recognise the possibility of the death of one's charge and, however reluctant one may be, this is a factor one really must not repress. Future social prospects must also be considered. If, through unremitting devotion to a patient, no other social contacts have been made or no other friendships maintained, the carer could be cutting off from associations which could be valuable in the future. And in the event of a bereavement, the situation is worse with no friends to offer consolation and sympathy.

DEALING WITH STRESS

Most people who accept responsibility for the care of a stroke patient suffer a continuously stressful life. Stress is a natural and necessary bodily response to the demands made upon it and the greater and more alarming the demands, the greater the stress. Sudden acute demands – such as the need to respond to serious danger – will produce an acute stress reaction with an outpouring of adrenaline and the body's own natural steroid to fuel the response. This is the well-known 'fright, fight or flight' reaction and with it we are able, sometimes, to perform wonders. Without these hormones we would be likely to come to grief. But if the hormones are not used as nature intended and we do not respond physically to the threat, the adrenaline and steroid simply rev up the engine and the result is severe anxiety. If this happens frequently, stress-related diseases like high blood pressure, duodenal ulcers and heart disease are likely.

Less severe demands, such as those experienced by the carer, still produce a definite stress reaction but, again, if the stress is not properly used or dissipated, the result will be a chronic state of fatigue and irritability with bad temper, anxiety, restlessness and often insomnia. The responsibility of attending to the wants of a stroke victim can be extremely stressful and most of the persistent factors causing this stress – physical exertion, mental perturbation, anxiety, frustration, resentment from various causes, and so on – have already been discussed. The effects are too well known to require more than mention. What is not well known is the proper way to handle this stress.

The first step is to recognise the stress and its effects and then take all reasonable measures to reduce it. Finally, because some measure of stress is unavoidable, one must learn how most effectively to live with it at minimum risk.

It is not difficult to recognise the presence of stress. Start by appreciating that the situation itself will almost certainly cause stress, then look for some of the following signs: a feeling of guilt, half-repressed anger, depression, a feeling of frustration, a sense of nagging insecurity, fatigue, insomnia, irritability, and an absence of calmness. These signs are unmistakeable and should not be ignored. Chronic stress is very bad and is liable to lead to ill-health or even a complete breakdown.

HOW TO REDUCE STRESS_____

The carer should carefully decide which of the many problems cause the most disturbance and annoyance. With Constance McLeod it was David's refusal to do anything for himself and his incontinence. Constance could not do much about the latter but she could, and did, make a tremendous effort to deal with, and overcome, the former. Of course, it will not always be possible to attack a central concern so directly as this and it will seldom be possible to get rid of it altogether. But, identifying the areas especially responsible for stress will put the carer in a position to examine them carefully and see what can be done to reduce their effect.

Whatever help other members of the family can give should be accepted gladly. If someone else can take over for a day, this may be a way of enlightening others about the size of the task, enlisting their sympathy and, hopefully, getting more help. One should always aim for a definite commitment to *regular*, weekly attendance. A day off once a week can work wonders and it is by no means unreasonable to expect help of this sort from other members of the family. No doubt there will be excuses, but if these are based on work responsibility, and the income from that work is fairly good, then there is no reason why one should not expect a financial contribution towards providing relief assistance.

Local authorities and welfare services may also be able to assist here. Full rights in state benefits should be obtained. Leaflets showing rights to attendance allowance, invalid care allowance, mobility allowance and so on are available. If in doubt as to entitlement, claim anyhow and if unfairly turned down, appeal. The best source of general information on these and many other matters which can substantially relieve a carer's stress, is the 'Directory for Disabled People' (a handbook of information and opportunities for disabled and handicapped people by Ann Darnborough and Derek Kinrade, published by Woodhead-Faulkner). This remarkable 360 page book, packed with useful information and advice, should be every carer's bible. The following American publications should also prove useful.

Catalog of Aids for the Disabled by Nancy and Jack Kreisler (McGraw-Hill 1982)

Bibliography on self-help devices by (National Easter Seal Society, 2023 West Ogden Avenue, Chicago, IL 60612)

Technology for Independent Living Resource Guide ed by Sandi Enders (RESNA, Suite 402, 4405 East-West Highway, Bethesda MD 20814)

Housing and Handicapped People by Marie M. Thompson (Available free from The President's Committee on Employment of the handicapped, Office of Publications, 1111 20th Street, Washington DC 20036 Tel 202-653-5157)

Access by Lilly Bruck (Random House 1978)

Advice on what is available in the way of technological and other aids is given in chapter 8 of this book, and one can decide whether any of these aids could make a contribution to stress reduction. Financial assistance can often be provided for these aids. For instance, it might make a major difference to the carer's stress, as well as greatly improving the quality of the patient's life, to have a stair lift installed giving access to both floors of a house. These lifts are expensive but wonderfully useful and most of the cost might be available from local authority funds.

Another way to reduce a cause of stress is to set priorities for responsibilities and, if necessary, allow some duties of lesser importance to go by default. A carer may be house proud and hate to see the place becoming dusty and the polish smeared. Well, in the context of increased duties, it may now be less damaging to health to allow standards to drop a little than to battle morning-to-night to maintain them. There may even be no one else to see how things are looking. Domestic pride can sometimes be an expensive luxury and one might be much better off with a new balance involving lowered standards and a little more time for much-needed rest and recreation.

Emotional reactions to the many frustrations and anxieties involved in caring duties should be watched. The catastrophe which has struck may have led the carer to wonder whether, and to what extent, he or she may have been responsible. This is a very common reaction, especially among wives of husbands who have had driving personalities. 'Was it my fault? Did I push him too hard by my extravagance or by my nagging demands for a better house or a bigger car? Was that row we had the cause of the stroke?'

This kind of reaction is natural and understandable but pointless, mistaken and damaging and should not be entertained for a moment. Strokes, are NOT caused by a flaming row or by a wife ambitious for social advancement.

Stress can be dissipated, or made less dangerous in several ways. One of these, surprisingly, is physical exercise but this should always be of a kind totally unconnected with the stressful situation. 'Fright, fight and flight' hormones have to be used up one way or another and the healthiest way to do this is by exercise. In younger people, this should be strenuous – squash, tennis, hard prolonged jogging, and so on – but in the more elderly, a quiet walk in a park or a sedate swim, done as a regular thing, can be most valuable. Formal relaxation can also be an effective way of dissipating stress. This has to be taken seriously and it may be a good idea to join an evening class in relaxation or Hatha Yoga so as to learn how to do it properly.

All measures to reduce stress will, in the end, benefit both carer and patient. The carer becomes a pleasanter person to live with, will tend to lose resentment, and will have more energy to devote to the many needs of the dependent charge.

STROKE CLUBS

One of the best ways of getting help is to arrange for the patient to join a stroke club. This will benefit both patient and carer in a number of ways, some of which have already been mentioned. If the patient is badly disabled the carer will probably also have to go to the club and this will give the opportunity for some badly-needed social activity and the chance to compare notes, and discuss problems, with the relatives of other stroke victims. Indeed, this aspect of stroke clubs has fostered 'Relative Support Groups', for the purpose of such discussions.

Stroke clubs have sprung up all over the country and there are now hundreds of them meeting usually once a month in local community centres or church halls. These, like other group activities for people with problems, have achieved a great deal more than might have been expected and it is now clear that the relatives almost invariably derive as much benefit as the patients. In a stroke club one meets others who have had exactly the same experience – people with the same burdens and anxieties – and some worse off. Other relatives share misfortunes, and are very pleased to give advice.

The emphasis in the majority of stroke clubs is on group support and friendly social activity. Members are encouraged to join in group games and competitions involving, for the benefit of people with aphasia, non-verbal activities such as chess, draughts, Mah Jong, dominoes and so on. Such games will often be played with great skill by those who are unable to read or speak. This is especially true if the person concerned was good at the game before the stroke occurred. Skills of this kind may sometimes be entirely unaffected even by severe strokes. But, in addition to the fun, there is also the serious purpose of educating both the stroke victim and members of the family in all aspects of the management of stroke. This is done both by informal discussion and by arranged lectures and talks by experts.

The social aspects of stroke clubs are a very important means of maintaining morale. Visits and outings of all kinds are regularly arranged so that stroke victims and their relatives may have a change of scene. Close friendships and valuable new relationships are frequently formed. Stroke clubs are considered to be one of the most encouraging and valuable developments in the management of stroke rehabilitation.

If difficulty is experienced in locating a nearby stroke club, write to The Chest Heart and Stroke Association, Tavistock House North, Tavistock Square, London WC1H 9JE. They keep a register of stroke clubs throughout the country and will be happy to advise. They also provide a great amount of literature for the guidance and help of carers (see page 114). Your local authority may well provide transportation to the club. Failing that, club officials keep a register of volunteer drivers who give their services as a social benefit.

The American equivalent of the Chest, Heart and Stroke Association is:

American Heart Association,
7320 Greenville Avenue,
Dallas, TX 75231
Tel 214-750-5551

This organisation maintains lists of stroke clubs and provides information services, exactly as the CHSA does. Another association, this one exclusively concerned with stroke, is the

National Stroke Association,
1565 Clarkson Street,
Denver, CO 80218
Tel 303-839-1992.

S-H

10 Sources of Help

People who have residual disability from stroke need all the help they can get and no book can possibly supply all the answers. This chapter outlines access to sources of information and guidance.

In Britain, the headquarters of the British Medical Association accommodates an organisation dedicated to the assistance of those who have suffered heart attacks and strokes. This is The Chest, Heart and Stroke Association, Tavistock House North, Tavistock Square, London WC1 9JE. For the equivalent organisations in the USA, please see pages 113 and 117–118. Any concerned person should certainly contact the CHSA if only with a view to discovering the address of the nearest stroke club. But encouraging the formation, and keeping a register of all stroke clubs in the country is by no means the limit of the CHSA's activities. The Association publishes a newspaper giving all sorts of news and advice to members and produces a number of very valuable booklets and pamphlets, primarily for the guidance of families of stroke patients. Some of these are:

Stroke. A Handbook for the Patient's Family
Stroke Illness – Twenty Questions and the Answers
Coping with Stroke Illness
Returning to Mobility
Learning to Speak Again
Reducing the Risk of Stroke
Facts about High Blood Pressure
Understanding Stroke Illness
Starting a Stroke Club – Twenty Questions and the Answers
Home Care for the Stroke Patient in the early Days
Our Games Book (Games for stroke patients)
A Time to Speak (Ideas for stroke patients with speech problems)
Hope – a Magazine of Optimism (Published quarterly)

The CHSA also produces cassettes to help improve the performance of those with speech problems, and a number of films and video tapes on stroke. The CHSA is active in supporting research on stroke, and sponsors 'The Volunteer Stroke Scheme' designed to help people with speech impairment. Under this scheme, volunteers, working with doctors and speech therapists, visit patients and organise clubs to help in speech rehabilitation.

An advisory service, which deals with over thirty thousand annual requests for help and advice, is another of the CHSA facilities and, in connection with this, the Association will even consider requests for financial assistance with fuel bills, rent and rate arrears, and costs of travelling to hospital. Since the CHSA is a voluntary organisation, dependent for its funds on charitable donations and bequests, money is limited, but in certain especially needful cases, assistance can be given.

Radar

The Royal Association for Disability and Rehabilitation, 25 Mortimer Street, London W1N 8AB, is a registered charity incorporating the British Council for Rehabilitation of the Disabled and the Central Council for the Disabled. Every month, except in September, the Association publishes a bulletin for disabled people, to keep them abreast of developments which might affect their lives. These bulletins, for which a small annual charge is made, deal with education, employment, mobility and access, holidays and relevant legislation. There is also a 'For Sale and Wanted' section. RADAR also publishes a quarterly magazine called *Contact* dealing with similar matters.

The Association's Publications List contains a large number of items, from fact sheets, costing a few pence, to complete books. Some are published by RADAR and others by various other authorities, but all can be ordered from the Association. A publication list is available on request. Here are some of the titles published by RADAR:

Holidays for Disabled People
Travelling with British Rail – a Guide for Disabled People
Holiday Factsheets (1–13)
Arts Centres (Facilities and amenities for the disabled)
The Countryside and Wildlife for Disabled People
Sports Centres for Disabled People
Sports and Leisure (An access guide for disabled spectators)
Get moving! (Transport for disabled people)
Mobility and Attendance Allowance

Mobility Factsheets (1–10)
Access to Public Conveniences
Area: Access and Means of Escape for Handicapped Employees
Building for the Disabled, 1981 Report
Choosing the best Wheelchair Cushion for your Needs, your Chair and your Lifestyle
Employability: Are you using your Assets?
Employers Guide to Disabilities
All Write Now (Journalism for disabled people)
Attitudes and Disabled People
The Handicapped Person

Other subjects covered include: access in overseas countries, at airports and at the Channel ports; medical costs abroad; Esso Service Station address list (stations whose operators are willing to help disabled people); lists of cinemas, theatres and entertainment halls in Greater London with facilities for disabled people; car choice; seat belts and the law; various other sheets on the law relating to the disabled; access guides to all main towns and cities; everyday aids for the disabled; notes on the use of gas and electricity; opportunities in microelectronics for disabled people; part-time employment; codes of practice for employers and other leaflets on employment published by the Manpower Services Commission; all aspects of housing relating to disabled people; legal and parliamentary provisions for the disabled; DHSS pamphlets concerning disabled people; communication aids for people with speech impairment; and many useful general reference books.

Most information needs are likely to be met from RADAR's impressive list of publications.

The Disabled Living Foundation

The Disabled Living Foundation, 380/384 Harrow Road, London W9 2HU has a large aids centre, where one may view, by appointment, a selection of aids to stroke patients. They also run a comprehensive information service which deals with over eighteen thousand individual enquiries a year and issues three and a half thousand bimonthly bulletins to subscribers. The information officers are qualified therapists experienced in the needs of disabled people and able to give excellent advice and guidance. The Foundation holds a very large central, computer-controlled information bank containing over twelve thousand references and keeps in close touch with research workers, manufacturers and suppliers of services so as to remain as up-to-date as possible. There is a large reference library which can be used by appointment. The telephone or letter enquiry service is open Monday to Friday from 9.30 AM to 5.00 PM.

The Disabled Living Foundation publishes many excellent pamphlets, notes and books, and provides information on many other books. Their information sheets cover such subjects as: aids for people who have had a stroke; beds suitable for hemiplegic and incontinent people; items to provide relief of pressure discomfort; chairs for disabled people; communication aids; eating and drinking aids; hoists and lifting equipment; leisure activities; sport for disabled people; personal toilet and personal care; transport; walking aids; manual and electric wheelchairs; household equipment; household fittings; incontinence aids; clothing; footwear; choosing a hoist; computer accessories; holiday information; adult and higher education; and many more.

Handicapped Living Monthly

This is an excellent monthly magazine published by A. E. Morgan Publications Ltd, Stanley House, 9 West Street, Epsom, Surrey KT18 7RT. The magazine's emphasis is on the fullest possible quality of life and deals with holidays, driving and mobility generally, advances in aids for the disabled, news and letters from disabled people, the use of computers by the disabled, and many other relevant matters. There are short stories, hobby articles, a crossword, and details of services for the disabled. The advertisements are also useful.

The USA

These are the important American organisations for handicapped individuals.

Office for Handicapped Individuals,
Room 338D, Hubert H. Humphrey Building,
200 Independence Avenue, SW,
Washington, DC 20201
Tel 202-245-1961

The National Council of Independent Living Programs,
4397 Laclede Avenue,
St Louis MO 63108
Tel 314-531-3050

Federation of the Handicapped,
211 West 14th Street,
New York NY 10011
Tel 212-242-9050

Rehabilitation International,
1123 Broadway,
New York NY 10010
Tel 212-620-4040

American Coalition of Citizens with Disabilities Inc,
Suite 201, 1200 15th Street NW,
Washington DC 20005
Tel 202-785-4265

There are over 200 Centers for Independent Living around the country. Consult your local white pages or telephone directories and call your nearest center. There you will find practical and emotional support, a warm welcome, and access to a great deal of vital information. You will get all the facts you need on the assistance available from city or county social service agencies and from private community organisations – things like funding for home modification; homemaking and chore services; aids; access; federal and local programs in aid of the disabled and much more.

Publications
Accent on Living – a quarterly magazine concerned with all ways of improving life for the disabled. PO Box 726, Bloomington, IL 61701

Rehabilitation Gazette – an annual journal and information service for disabled people. Contains full lists of US periodicals and newsletters for the disabled. 4502 Maryland Avenue, St Louis, MO 63108 Tel 314-361-0475

The Institute of Rehabilitation Medicine,
400 East 34th Street,
New York NY 10016

This organisation offers many publications on the rehabilitation of the disabled.

Sources of equipment and aids for the disabled

SH Camp and Company,
PO Box 89,
Jackson MI 49204

J. A. Preston Corporation,
71 Fifth Avenue,
New York NY 10003

G. E. Miller Inc,
484 South Broadway,
Yonkers, NY 10705

Rehabilitation Equipment Inc,
1556 Third Avenue,
New York NY 10028

Nelson Medical Products,
5690 Sarah Avenue,
Sarasota FL 33581

J. T. Posey Company,
39 South Santa Anita Avenue,
Pasadena CA 91107

Rehabilitation Equipment
and Supply,
1823 West Moss Avenue,
Peoria IL 61606

Self-Help Equipment Firms,
Cleo Living Aids,
3957 Mayfield,
Cleveland OH 44121

Australia

The directory of stroke clubs is kept by The Australian Council for Rehabilitation of the Disabled, Acrod House, 33 Thesiger Court, Deakin, South Australia. A feature of rehabilitation in Australia is the establishment, in most states, of 'Independent Living Centres' dedicated to the preservation, whenever possible, of personal independence. Here is a list of these Centres:

New South Wales PO Box 351, 277 Morrison Road, Ryde, 2112
Queensland   Ward 1, Repatriation General Hospital, Newdegate Street, Green Slopes, 4120
Victoria   PO Box 3025, 52 Thistlethwaite Street, South Melbourne, 3205
South Australia 40 Cheltenham Street, Highgate, 5063
West Australia PO Box 257, 5 Lemnos Street, Shenton Park, 6008

Other helpful books

Two very useful and comprehensive books have been written by Ann Darnborough and Derek Kinrade. These dedicated writers on assistance for the disabled have compiled two remarkable directories, both published by Woodhead-Faulkner Ltd. They are:

Directory for Disabled People (4th edition, 1985)

This is an amazingly detailed handbook of information for disabled people, covering every aspect of disability. Subjects include: statutory services for the disabled; financial benefits and allowances; the provision and availability of aids for the disabled; statutory provisions, grants and allowances for the home; education; employment; motoring and mobility; holidays at home and abroad; sports and leisure activities; sex and personal relationships; legislation affecting the disabled; organisations; and information, legal and advisory services.

This list gives little indication of the wealth of information in this invaluable book, much of which will be of value to people who have suffered disability of one sort or another as a result of stroke.

Directory of Aids for Disabled and Elderly People (1986)

This equally remarkable book shows the surprising lengths to which ingenious people have gone to improve the quality of life of the disabled. Here is a positive mine of information on thousands of ways in which people can be helped to overcome their physical and personal problems.

Every aspect of life in which aids can be helpful is dealt with and the book covers such diverse subjects as entitlement to relief from VAT; car tax and import duty on aids to the disabled; communication; clothing; incontinence; wheelchairs and wheelchair accessories; hoists; slings and lifts; walking and standing aids; motoring and motoring with a wheelchair; kitchen and household aids; bathroom aids and aids to personal hygiene; toilet aids; living room and bedroom aids; aids for sports and leisure and gardening aids. There are many advertisements and a very full appendix giving manufacturers, addresses and telephone numbers.

Books for further information

Other books can be recommended to those avid for information. One of the best known is *Stroke. A Diary of Recovery* by Douglas Ritchie and published by Faber and Faber. In clear, dramatic fashion, it tells the story of the experience of a busy professional man, head of a department at the BBC, who suffered a severe stroke. It recounts his struggle to recover from hemiplegia and speech impairment and describes his hopes, fears and disappointments in a very matter-of-fact and readable manner. This is a human, honest and inspiring account and should be studied by every stroke patient able to do so.

Valerie Eaton Griffiths helped Patricia Neal recover her speech after a series of strokes, using a method developed by herself. Called *A Stroke in the Family* this is an excellent little work which outlines the method she used in helping both Miss Neal and Alan Moorehead, the famous writer and historian. It is thoroughly recommended. Published by Wildwood House in 1970.

Return to Mobility by Margaret Hawker and Amanda Squires, published by the Chest, Heart and Stroke Association, is a splendidly written and admirably illustrated account of exercises and procedures designed to ensure maximal recovery. It covers every activity of normal living and gives much excellent advice. It is a strongly bound publication and very good value for money.

Learning to Speak Again after a Stroke by Charles R. Isted is published by the King Edward's Hospital Fund for London, 126 Albert Street, London

NW1 7NF. Charles Isted is a professional Engineer who describes his recovery of speech after a stroke. The book is printed in very large type and contains lists of practice words and eighteen exercises, with answers.

Other useful books for the non-medical reader are:

Help Yourself (4th edition 1985) by Peggy Jay sponsored by RADAR and CHSA.

Incontinence by Dorothy Mandelstam (Disabled Living Foundation)

Coping with Disability by Peggy Jay (Disabled Living Foundation)

Entitled to Love by Wendy Greengross (Malaby Press)

Computer Help for Disabled People by Lorna Ridgway and Stuart McKears (Souvenir Press – Human Horizons Series)

Books on rehabilitation

Several books dealing with the medical aspects of the rehabilitation of stroke victims, have been published, but most of these are not specifically intended for lay consumption and may make difficult reading. Nevertheless, there is much of value in these books and some of them are written by dedicated nurses and occupational therapists who are dissatisfied with the present standards of medical care following stroke.

Restoration of Motor Function in the Stroke Patient by Margaret Johnstone (Churchill Livingstone, 2nd edition, 1983). This is really a textbook for physiotherapists but is full of detail based on sound medical principles and should be very useful to the more enquiring layman.

Nursing Care of the Hemiplegic Stroke Patient by Freda Myco, (Harper & Row 1983). Again, this book may present some difficulties to the non-medical reader, but it provides a comprehensive account of the management of stroke-paralysed people and deals, thoroughly, with posture and mobility; nutrition; elimination; personal hygiene; sleep and rest; communication; sexuality; leisure and employment and spiritual matters.

Practical Management of Stroke by Graham P. Mulley (Croom Helm 1985) is a book for medical professionals but is an extremely clear and practical account of the subject, written with unusual humanity. It contains a useful chapter on the problems of the relatives of stroke victims. Up to now, most of the emphasis on rehabilitation of stroke patients has been found in books by occupational therapists, physiotherapists and nurses. The matter has been relatively neglected by the medical profession and Dr Mulley does much in this book to challenge the common medical assumption that comparatively little can be done for stroke patients. This excellent book is written in technical language and will make difficult reading.

11 Coming to Terms with Permanent Disability

MAKING A VIRTUE OF NECESSITY_____

Coming to terms with a disability is a battle that the sufferer fights alone. Decisions have to be made about the direction of future life, and courage and resources have to be found to reach a point where one can say 'Well, life isn't so bad, after all.' Happily, there are many ways in which patients can be helped to reach this point and much effort has been expended, by many devoted people, to ease the way. This chapter is addressed to the stroke victim, to bring to his, or her attention some of the many ways of coming to terms with disability.

Sufferers from stroke illness should not think themselves unique. There are plenty of other people in the same situation and many worse off. About twenty per cent of people who have had strokes, and survive, are never able to return home. Most of the others show some degree of recovery. Thirty per cent are able to resume a fairly normal life and about ten per cent show no outward sign of any problem. But about half of the people who suffer strokes every year end up with significant permanent physical or mental incapacity. Indeed, stroke is the largest single cause of severe permanent disability.

The stages in the psychological reactions to the effects of stroke have been covered in Chapter 5. We must now consider the later stages when further recovery is unlikely and it is apparent that there are going to be permanent effects. Hopefully a high standard of occupational, physio- and speech therapy has achieved maximal recovery in walking and speech. But now that these stages are past and physical adaptation is as complete as it is likely to be, what happens now? The real question is how best to make a virtue of necessity. The aim, first and last, must be to live life to the full and, if humanly possible, to achieve more than had been expected before the stroke occurred.

This may seem paradoxical and asking rather a lot, but the suggestion is put forward with full seriousness. The great majority of healthy people waste much of their lives and never realise a fraction of their potential.

The change of lifestyle, the more sedentary and restricted life imposed by disability may, if there is sufficient determination, concentrate attention and unrealised abilities into new and more productive channels, and the result may be surprising.

The worst thing to do is to remain aggrieved, sorry for oneself and bitter. If the remainder of life is not to be ruined, one simply must turn and look outwards, cultivate appropriate new and absorbing interests and drive them to the limit. One must learn to work harder than ever before – to forget about rest – it's not necessary – and get absorbed in something new, creative and fascinating. Something like running an accountancy business from a wheel-chair; managing an agency; taking a degree; writing new computer software; engaging in modem communication with the rest of the world; working to qualify for an amateur radio licence or getting into CB radio; taking up oil, water-colour or acrylic painting; mosaic creation; stained glass window construction; writing biographies, fiction, specialised non-fiction, magazine articles.

Perhaps none of these things is appealing. Or it may be that, for years, despite a hankering to be a writer or a painter or a computer programmer, nothing has been done about it because of lack of spare time. It makes no difference either way. The reasons for taking up an absorbing new occupation, now, are very serious. Much too serious to be brushed casually aside because of mere disinclination or apparent lack of interest. It is important to recognise that interest is a commodity of priceless value and that it will come only with deliberate indulgence in new activity, growing knowledge and experience. Interest can grow to fascination. Interest displaces misery, self-preoccupation, boredom, depression. Contentment is a matter of filling the mind with a concern that constantly prompts curiosity.

There is going to be a great deal of time to spend – and time can be a curse or a blessing depending on whether or not one has something to do with it. The object must now be so to fill the mind with interest that there are simply not enough hours in the day.

In addition to the sudden access of leisure time, the new circumstances are, inevitably, going to make it more difficult to keep up with many old friends. This is an unfortunate fact of disabled life that one must learn to accept. Some few may be faithful but, to the severely physically disabled, the majority of acquaintances are almost certainly lost for ever. So, one must find new friends and the way to do this is to establish real interests and then proceed to seek out those who share them. Some of the activities mentioned have the means of doing this built in. The development of cheap electronic and computer technology has brought communication possibilities of unprecedented scope within reach, allowing extension of personal range of contact. Writing, too, both private and public, has been made very much easier, as we shall see shortly. Again, people who attend evening or day adult education classes, whether disabled or not, have a common interest. Except in remote areas, classes are available in an extremely wide range of subjects.

It would be wrong to imply that all post-stroke activity has to be sedentary. Most stroke sufferers are at an age at which they would, in any case, have begun to settle down to a physically less active life. But some may have been accustomed to sporting activity and this may have been very important to them. Unless one is seriously disabled, there is often scope for continuing to engage in sport of one kind or another. Depending on the type and degree of disability, this may be either as a participant or as a spectator. One should not be too pessimistic about this. There are many inspiring examples of almost incredible feats of athleticism and skill among those who have suffered the kind of physical disability common after stroke.

Some may be tempted to try to pass the time by playing simple games, reading light fiction and watching video films. While there is, of course, a place for unchallenging games and passive entertainment, and these may be the only resources for those whose mental powers are affected by stroke, it is a great mistake for the mentally active to think that time can be satisfactorily filled by such means. Time must not be regarded as something to be disposed of, and if this is how the patient regards it then he or she is already in trouble and badly needs the advice contained in this Chapter. There are games, such as chess or bridge, which may challenge one's mental resources to the limit and these may be, or may become, an absorbing part-time activity.

Life-enhancement by computer

We have seen how the microcomputer can be used as to aid direct communication within the household for those with speech disablement. Wider applications exist and the absence of a technical background should not prevent anyone from making excellent use of computers. They may be thought of as 'black boxes' in which something mysterious happens when one touches certain keys, the result being a useful output of some kind, either on the screen or at the printer. Pressing the wrong keys may cause problems and may waste work already done, but cannot harm the computer.

Word processing

Nowadays the great majority of word processors are ordinary microcomputers fed with a suitable word processing program, and most of these do everything that the older dedicated machines could do, at a small fraction of the price. It is important that the micro chosen should have a proper, high quality, keyboard and, ideally, a number of so-called 'function' keys.

Many people think that a word processor is a complicated device, very difficult to master, but this is simply not true. One reason for including the subject here is that a word processor is, in fact, very much easier to use than a typewriter – especially for a disabled person. The one-handed typist, struggling with a standard electric typewriter has major problems. Mistakes are inevitable, corrections are difficult – especially with carbon paper – spoiled paper is awkward to replace and editorial changes are so tedious to make that one is likely to leave the work in a less than perfect state.

With a word processor, nearly all these difficulties are eliminated. Everything typed on the keyboard appears first on a screen and the effect of any additions, deletions or alterations is immediately visible there. The required key pressure is light; 'carriage return' occurs automatically at the end of each line; margins can be set, as desired, from the keyboard; type can be justified at will; mistakes are corrected on the screen quite simply, either by overtyping or by deleting and inserting new letters or words; and the most detailed editing can be done at the touch of a few keys. Words, sentences, paragraphs, or even pages of type can be shifted around until everything is exactly right. Only then need the printing be done, by a simple keyboard command. The shift key, and shift lock (for capital letters) require no more force than any other key and this is a great help when using the left hand. Because corrections are so easy, one is encouraged to work boldly and will soon achieve good speed, even with one hand.

At any time, the work can be saved on disks, to be added to, or printed, later. These disks can hold an immense amount of material – with the more sophisticated machines a whole book can be stored on one or two disks and they can be kept for years, for future reference or revision. Any word processing microcomputer can be connected to a 'daisy-wheel' printer that will produce superb typescript to rival that of the finest electric typewriter, and at considerably less cost. There is no end to the possibilities of the word processor for anyone with writing ambitions, and countless disabled people bless the day they were introduced to this remarkable application of modern microelectronics.

A recent development is home electronic book production. At the time of writing, this calls for equipment costing a few thousand pounds, but the possibilities are remarkable. It is now feasible to produce complete books – to carry out all the functions of the writer, the illustrator, the editor, the proof-reader, the designer – indeed the whole writing and publishing function, except for printing and distribution, in the privacy of one's own home. 'Camera ready' copy of each page is produced on disk, which can then go straight to the printer for mass reproduction. The same can be done, just as easily, for magazines of all kinds, and it is even possible to get contributors to send their copy direct into your computer, for editing and arrangement, by telephone line. With ideas, writing, artistic and design ability, anybody could be the producer of a money-making magazine within a month or two.

The keyboard emulator

Most stroke patients have the use of at least one hand and this allows very effective word processing using standard equipment. There are some, however, who, while retaining full intellectual power, are very severely disabled physically, and may not even have independent finger use on one side. Happily, even to these, the benefits of computer use may still be available with an additional facility which displays, on part of the screen, or, in the more sophisticated versions, on a separate screen, a complete keyboard layout, duplicating the real keyboard.

It is then possible using a small 'joystick' switch, to cause a highlighted indicator (the cursor) to move about the displayed keyboard to indicate the required letters or functions. These may then be definitively selected by pressing the joystick button, and the effect is exactly as if a key on the actual keyboard had been pressed. All this may sound dreadfully cumbersome and slow, but it is really remarkable how much speed can be achieved with practice. Keyboard emulators come in a variety of forms and there are even some that can be used by totally paralysed people, operated by a 'blow – suck' switch, a head-supported spot-light, or even eye movements or the sound of the voice.

The MODEM

Another important application of the microcomputer for disabled people is remote communication. There is no practical limit to this, and the possession of a microcomputer, a telephone connection and some minor ancillary equipment allows link up to any other computer in the world. Whatever is typed on the screen can be transmitted and it is possible to receive from any other computer, whatever a known password allows. Nowadays, the great majority of computers have a socket on the back known as a 'serial port' (sometimes called an RS 232 'interface') and those not so equipped can always be fitted with such a connection. The purpose of the serial port is to convert the form of the data, held within the computer, to a common form so as to enable the micro to be linked with any other computer having a serial port. Because all data is converted to a simple common form, this is possible whatever the make or type of the machines used.

The information leaving one's computer in standard serial form, consists of a rapid succession of two different electrical levels and, in order to be conveyed reliably by telephone lines, has to be converted into the electrical equivalent of actual sounds suitable for transmission by telephone. At the other end, these signals are changed back into electrical levels identical to those sent out. These changes, from electrical to acoustical, and back again, are described as 'MOdulation' and 'DEModulation' and the fairly simple gadget that does this is, reasonably enough, called a MODEM. They have been in use for many years by telephone engineers, but it is only in the last few years that it has become commonplace for them to be used by ordinary people in their own homes.

Accessing the databases

The possession of a simple microcomputer and a MODEM together with the necessary program (communications software) to instruct the computer to send whatever is in its memory out at the serial port and to accept and store incoming messages, opens up a whole new world. It is possible, for instance, to access data banks of information, both in Britain and abroad. These banks are called databases, and the sheer size of them and the range of subjects covered, beggar the imagination.

DIALOG, for instance, is the largest store of electronically accessible information in the world, including subjects as diverse as agriculture, geology, biology, drugs, economics, the environment, food science, investment, language, law, mathematics, medicine, pollution, psychology, sociology, stock markets, trademarks, who's who, world affairs and zoology. On many of these subjects there are several – sometimes as many as ten – separate databases, and DIALOG is only one of the many vast stores of information accessible in this way. A system called the 'Knowledge Index' provides British subscribers with low-cost access to the most popular databases on DIALOG during British off-peak hours, so that one is actually in connection with the main storage computers in California for a fraction of the cost of a transatlantic telephone call. Information is passed at a tremendous speed and, although the rate is almost £20 per hour, since only a few minutes will be spent actually on line, the total cost, unless one gets completely carried away, will be very small.

Datasbases are constantly updated and the amount of information contained in them is staggering. All this is available on demand, for a reasonable subscription and the cost of the telephone call. The information needed will appear on the screen of the microcomputer and can be stored on disks and, if necessary, printed out as 'hard copy'.

Computer graphics

This is a fascinating new departure with wide applications for people who are disabled. Forget the crude, garish novelty computer displays in shop windows. Modern graphics software works to a high degree of resolution with an almost infinite range of colours, and offers the artistically-inclined disabled person astonishing control and scope for imagination. The best modern graphics software allows complex manipulation of shapes and areas, with controlled distortion and rotation into any plane, automatic colouring of areas, however large or small, and enlargement or reduction at will. The possibilities are unlimited.

Several commercial machines exist which enable the immediate production of 35mm slides from the finished design so that ready copy can go straight off to the publisher. Alteration and additions, lettering, in any typeface, and adjustment to the outline dimensions, perhaps to suit the publisher's requirements, can easily be made. It seems inevitable that the computer-aided approach to artwork will become standard and the disabled will be able to compete, almost on equal terms, with the unafflicted. A whole new, and perhaps highly paid, career may be opened up to disabled people with the appropriate artistic and design abilities. These are the talents required, *not* technical know-how.

The on-line office

This development should be of central interest to those whose business or commercial career has been cut short by a stroke. A growing number of firms – accountancy, sales, real estate, public relations, advertising – are beginning to appreciate that it is extremely cost effective for as many employees as possible to work in their own homes. Using computer communications, the link with employees is as complete as if they were physically present in the office.

Although still in its infancy, this trend is growing rapidly. It will be a positive boon to the physically disabled but intellectually unimpaired business person who may be able to enjoy an unrestricted business career, including promotion, without moving out of the home. Rank

Xerox have been trying out the idea in the last few years and their experience has been described in a book 'Networking in Organisations – the Rank Xerox Experiment' (Phillip Judkins, David West and John Drew, published by Gower Publishing, 1986). This book recounts how more than fifty Rank Xerox employees moved from their offices back to their homes, and contains personal accounts of the experience of several of them. It also deals with the principles of 'networking' and the selection and training of employees for this purpose.

One should not be put off by the seemingly alarming technology involved. It is not necessary to be an electronic engineer to use a TV set or a video tape recorder. Operating a computer terminal has been mastered by many thousands of people much less able than many stroke victims and is simply a matter of a little practice. What really counts is business experience, judgement and capacity for hard work.

Other computer applications

This is a very large subject inappropriate to explore much further in this book. But what has been said may encourage stroke patients to look into the possibilities themselves. The literature available is now enormous. Those with business and accounting skills will probably already be familiar with computer applications, but will want to see whether they can now apply their experience even more effectively by means of modern accounting software. Packages of programs covering all aspects of business management and offering ways of improving efficiency, cash flow and profitability are now available from scores of different software houses, for all standard microcomputers.

An important development is the growth of data base management systems – programs which enable the user, after accumulating data, to access items in almost any way desired. A number of major programs of this type, designed to allow custom building of a system for special requirements, have been produced. Programs like dBase II, dBase III, Delta and others enable one, without writing actual program code, to produce software to exact needs. It is even possible to do this for other people as a profit-making activity.

Spread sheets, report generators, statistics programs, stock market programs, money managers, general ledgers, tax accounting programs, management system, desk organisers, decision makers, computer-aided design systems, educational programs of all kinds, programs on programming – the list is endless and the variety, in each of these categories, amazing. Novices should begin carefully and start by checking exactly what an apparently suitable item of software will do, and confirm that that

S-I

is exactly what is needed. Having settled on the software, one should think about which computer to buy, comparing prices and ensuring that the software will run on the machine you are considering. Claims that a given machine is 'compatible' with one which runs the chosen software should be treated with caution. In the micro world, the word 'compatible' is a very relative term. It is always best to insist on a full demonstration of the program before parting with money.

For these purposes 8 bit machines are now obsolete as they can only handle a limited (64 Kilobyte) memory. A 16 bit machine that will run MS-DOS or CP/M (disc operating systems) is needed. Note that storing data on cassettes is far too slow. 8 bit machines are very cheap and are fine for home communications but they are not really any good for serious business purposes.

Computer applications can be very creative, and it is a pity, since computers can do so much for disabled people, that many people find computers unattractive. However, there are many more equally engrossing interests to develop, often artistic ones, such as sketching, watercolour, oil and acrylic painting, tile making, crockery decoration, tapestry, fine sewing and embroidery, knitting and weaving.

SKETCHING AND PAINTING

In following artistic pursuits of this kind, much advice and helpful encouragement can be obtained from 'Conquest – The Art Society for the Physically Handicapped', 3 Beverley Close, East Ewell, Epsom, Surrey KT17 3HB. The object of Conquest is to encourage people with physical handicaps to take up and become involved in creative artistic activity. Conquest publishes a magazine and various helpful pamphlets, and the groups belonging to the organisation hold exhibitions from time to time.

Severe muscle weakness is, of course, always a problem, and various supports are available. These can be attached to work tables, benches and wheelchairs. One of the most versatile systems, the Orange Aids System, is produced by Hugh Steeper (Roehampton) Ltd, 237-239 Roehampton Lane, London SW15 4LB. This consists of a range of adjustable clamps, grips, vices and mobile arm supports, which can be attached to almost anything. These give the necessary positioning for the use of very weak arms and hands, while appropriately locating the boards or canvas for painting or sketching or frames for embroidery. The Steeper system also includes scissors attachments, which can be operated by hand or foot, glass holders, mirrors, adjustable magnifying glasses and lecterns. Writers who feel happier with the traditional pen or pencil rather than with a word processor can also benefit from this system.

GARDENING

Gardening is immensely popular and is a great source of satisfaction to people disabled by stroke. Whether or not it will be possible to sustain the former level of activity will depend on the severity of the disability, but, at worst, and with the assistance of good advice and the support of one or other of the organisations concerned with gardening for the disabled, it should certainly be possible to maintain some interest and pleasure. Perhaps the size of the garden or allotment will have to be limited or interests changed to the cultivation of more exotic conservatory or greenhouse flora. Possibly the patient may even have to think in terms of large window boxes or simply indoor plants, but it is unlikely that the interest will have to be given up altogether.

Gardening on a reasonably large scale may be ambitious but is certainly better than unnecessary limitation. Heavy work may seem impossible but, again, technology can assist. This is not because of the existence of any special gardening aids for the disabled, but simply because gardening has become such big business that many tools and gadgets have been developed to make the work easier for the ordinary, able-bodied person. Working from a wheel-chair calls for tools to extend the reach and there are plenty of these. Items intended for one job can, with imagination, be adapted for another. Fruit pickers and long tongs can considerably extend the range of activities. These are available in lengths of from four to ten feet and some can be operated by one hand.

There are branch cutters with considerable leverage and a rachet action which require remarkably little strength; various grabbers and long-handled weeders, capable of one-handed use, some designed to grip and pull out the most stubborn weeds; wheelrakes which do not have to be lifted in use; ingenious hoes (for example the 'multihoe') which can perform a variety of operations very easily; lightweight lawn shears with long handles for edging and general grass cutting; lightweight wheel-barrows; electric trimmers and hedge cutters (not for the one-handed!) and many other useful gadgets. A visit to a large garden centre and a study of the garden tool section should pay dividends.

Those confined to a wheelchair might consider a garden in raised pots or even complete raised flower beds. The latter are available in reinforced concrete, galvanised steel or fibreglass and come in a wide range of sizes, some with preserved timber exteriors. Seating can be arranged around these raised beds. A herb garden would be one idea.

Help can be obtained from organisations such as the Gardens for the Disabled Trust, Church Cottage, Headcorn, Kent TN27 9NP. This organisation provides information and advice on all matters relating to gardening for the disabled. Similarly, the Garden Research Department of the Nuffield Orthopaedic Centre, Mary Marlborough Lodge, Headington, Oxford OX3 7LD will gladly answer queries if a stamped, self-addressed envelope is sent. The Research Department has a programme of investigation into the best ways of helping disabled gardeners to enjoy the activity.

The Society for Horticultural Therapy and Rural Training, Goulds Ground, Vallis Way, Frome, Somerset BA11 3DW is another enterprise offering an information service for disabled people, and has a training centre running courses of instruction for those working with disabled people. It publishes an excellent magazine called *Growth Point* of great interest to all disabled people interested in gardening.

Some books and pamphlets on gardening for the physically handicapped are:

The Easy Path to Gardening (Reader's Digest in conjunction with the Disabled Living Foundation).

Gardening for the Disabled – a set of papers with lists of suitable tools and plans for raised flower beds (Disabled Living Foundation).

Gardening for the Physically Handicapped and Elderly (Mary Chaplin, B. T. Batsford Ltd, 4 Fitzhardinge Street, London W1H 0AH).

Gardening is for Everyone; A Week-by-Week Guide for People with Handicaps (Audrey Cloet and Chris Underhill, Souvenir Press Ltd, 43 Great Russell Street, London WC1B 3PA).

Leisure and Gardening This is one of a series entitled *Equipment for the Disabled* and is available from the Nuffield Orthopaedic Centre, Mary Marlborough Lodge, Headington, Oxford OX3 7LD.

12 Glossary

Adrenaline A powerful chemical agent produced by small glands on top of each kidney, in response to emergency situations. It raises the blood pressure, increases the heart rate and prepares the body for violent action.

Alexia The loss of the ability to understand written or printed words.

Aneurysm A local ballooning of an artery. There is risk of rupture with severe bleeding. Aneurysms often occur on brain arteries and rupture is one of the causes of stroke. (*See* subarachnoid haemorrhage).

Aphasia Inability to speak or to understand spoken language. A common effect of stroke. It often occurs as a transient effect following a stroke, but is sometimes permanent. (*See* dysphasia)

Apoplexy An old-fashioned name for stroke. It was usually applied to cerebral haemorrhage.

Artery A blood vessel conveying blood under pressure from the heart to remote parts of the body. Disease of the arteries is the cause of stroke. (*See* atherosclerosis, vein).

Atherosclerosis The commonest cause of death. A disease of the inner linings of arteries in which cholesterol, fats and other substances are deposited. This narrows the vessels and reduce the amount of blood which can pass.

Body image The idea, or image, one has of the shape and appearance of one's own body. Body image can be affected by stroke, both by awareness of paralysis and by loss of sensation on one side. An impaired body image can interfere with recovery.

Brainstem The narrowed, lower part of the brain, just above the spinal cord. The brainstem contains vital centres for the maintenance of breathing and heart action, an elaborate set of nerve connections concerned with facial expression, eye movement and balance, and many other important structures. Severe stroke affecting the brainstem is usually fatal.

CT scan (CAT scan) Computer assisted tomography. A very advanced form of X-ray in which the signals from a long sequence of separate, low-power, narrow-beam radiation scans are put together by computer to form a detailed image. CT scan can show areas of brain damaged by stroke. Recent generation machines can show very fine detail.

Cardiovascular Concerning the heart and the blood vessels.

Carotid artery One of a pair of vital arteries supplying the head and brain with blood. The carotids run up the front of the neck and maintain the supply to the middle and front half of the brain, as well as the face and scalp. Carotid artery disease is one of the main causes of stroke. (*See* vertebral artery).

Cerebral cortex The outer layer of the main, upper part of the brain. The cortex can be mapped out into areas which are the highest physical representation of the functions of intellect, movement, sensation, hearing, speech, vision and so on.

Cerebral haemorrhage Bleeding, from a burst artery, into the substance of the brain or into the surrounding areas within the skull. This is, in general, the most serious cause of stroke. Cerebral haemorrhage often occurs within an area containing the main nerve fibres concerned with movement.

Cerebral oedema Swelling of the brain substance. This occurs around damaged areas and causes a loss of function which is often only temporary.

Cerebral thrombosis The closing off, by blood clotting, of any artery supplying part of the brain with blood. This is a very common cause of stroke. (*See* atherosclerosis).

Cerebro-vascular accident (CVA) A medical euphemism for stroke. It is not a very good phrase as strokes are hardly ever accidental.

Cerebrum The main, upper part of the brain. It consists of two cerebral hemispheres, joined together and containing the parts by which memory, intellect and emotion are subserved; movement, locomotion and speech initiated; vision and all forms of sensation experienced; language understood; and artistic and creative activity undertaken. These parts lie mainly on the surface (the cerebral cortex) and are joined with each other, and with deeper brain structures, by massive bundles of nerve fibres. Any of these parts may be damaged in the course of a stroke.

Cholesterol A steroid alcohol found in animal fats and eggs. It is a normal body constituent, but high cholesterol in the diet and in the bloodstream may contribute to disease of the arteries. (*See* atherosclerosis).

Circle of Willis The important circle of arteries at the base of the brain into which branches of both the carotid and the vertebral arteries run, and by which means the supply to the brain is made more secure.

Coma A state of deep unconsciousness. The affected person cannot be awakened and shows no response to stimuli which would normally be painful, Severe stroke often causes coma and many patients die without recovering consciousness.

Coronary artery One of the two vital arteries coming from the main arterial trunk immediately above the heart, and supplying the heart muscle itself with blood. (*See* coronary thrombosis)

Coronary thrombosis Blockage, by clotting, of one of the coronary arteries or one of their branches. This is usually the result of atherosclerosis and is always serious. Non-fatal coronary thrombosis can lead to the development of clots on the inner heart lining and these can be carried up to the brain to cause stroke.

Cortisol The natural steroid hormone. Essential to life, but excessive production, along with adrenaline, in stressful situations, can be harmful.

Depression Sadness, discouragement and despair. A state of mourning resulting from some personal loss, bereavement or tragedy. May also occur without external cause, as a disorder of the mind. Depression is almost universally experienced by people who have had strokes and it may impede recovery.

Disability The loss of power, function or learned skill of either body or mind. Disability is the usual long-term effect of stroke and may vary from the most trifling to the most extreme. The commonest major disabilities following stroke are hemiplegia and dysphasia. (q.v.)

Dysphasia A less than complete disturbance of the communication function. There may be disturbance of speech or understanding of language, or both.

Embolism When a blood clot, or other material lying within a blood vessel, is moved by the blood-stream, from its site of origin to a narrower part or branch, of the vessel, blockage occurs. Such movement and blockage is called an embolism, and the material causing the blockage is called an embolus. Embolism is a common cause of TIAs and stroke. (*See* transient ischaemic attacks).

Emotional lability A condition of emotional instability in which the mood of the person swings rapidly from one state to another – from joy to sorrow, from affection to anger, and so on. Sometimes the expression of the emotion is inappropriate or extreme.

Haemorrhage Bleeding.

Hemianopia A common effect of stroke in which half of the field of vision of each eye is lost. This may be both right or both left halves. This happens because of the way the optic nerves are connected to the brain.

Hemiplegia Loss of the power of movement in one half of the body. The right half of the brain controls the left half of the body and vice versa. Since stroke nearly always affects one half of the brain only, hemiplegia is very common.

Hypertension Abnormally high blood pressure.

Impotence The inability to obtain, or maintain, a penile erection and so perform full sexual intercourse. The commonest cause, even after stroke, is psychological disturbance, usually anxiety about potency.

Incontinence Loss of control over the urinary bladder or bowel action, so that urine or faeces are discharged spontaneously at inconvenient times. This may be a result of stroke, but recovery is common.

Ischaemia The state of a tissue whose blood supply has been reduced or cut off. This is caused by disease of the arteries supplying the part, usually atherosclerosis. Ischaemia of part of the brain is a very common cause of stroke.

Motor nerve A nerve connected to a muscle. The nerve impulse causes the muscle to shorten and movement to result.

Reflex An action – often a movement – which occurs involuntarily as a result of a stimulus. A muscle, paralysed by stroke, will commonly go into spasm, by reflex action, as a result of stretching or other stimulus.

Sensory nerve A nerve carrying information about touch, pain, temperature, etc, from the skin, or from an internal organ, inwards to the nervous system. Sensory connections to the brain can be affected by stroke and the result is a loss of the particular sensations carried.

Sexuality The totality of the physical, mental and functional characteristics of one's gender. Sexuality involves far more than simply a concern about physical sexual relations.

Spasm Involuntary contraction of a muscle. May be prolonged and painful. Spasm is always disabling and may cause disfigurement. It must be avoided if the fullest recovery after stroke is to be achieved.

Spastic paralysis Loss of voluntary movement, with involuntary contraction of muscles on stretching. This is very typical of hemiplegia following stroke.

Stimulus Anything that excites a response.

Stroke in evolution An unfortunate situation in which disability increases step by step. This progression may go on for up to two weeks, when the full extent of the disability will be clear.

Sub-arachnoid haemorrhage A bleeding between the brain surface and one of the covering membranes. Typically caused by a ruptured aneurysm. This is a common cause of stroke, often in younger people.

Subtraction imaging arteriography A recent, and highly refined, form of investigation of artery disease in which two computer imaging pictures are taken, an X-ray opaque dye being injected into the blood-stream between them. One picture is then turned into a negative and the two superimposed. Identical features cancel out leaving the image of the dye in the vessels. This can show up atherosclerosis, aneurysms and other diseases.

TIA (Transient Ischaemic Attack) A brief episode, like a stroke in miniature, caused by temporary shutting off of blood to a part of the brain. Any of the effects of stroke may occur, but only briefly. TIAs are warnings of impending stroke and should *never* be disregarded.

Vein A thin-walled blood vessel carrying blood, at low pressure, from the remote parts of the body back towards the heart.

Vertebral Artery One of a pair of important vessels running up the neck within the bones of the spine and supplying the back half of the brain with blood. (*See* carotid artery).

Index

Adrenaline, 60, 132
Aids for stroke patients, 90, 91
  bathroom, 92, 93
  kitchen, 90
  sitting room, 91
Alexia, 133
Amerind, 79
Aneurysm, 29, 133
  double vision from, 29
  headache from, 29
  stroke and, 31
Aorta, 11
Aphasia, 10, 39
  cause, 70
  psychotherapy, 80
  types, 71, 77
Apoplexy, 29, 32, 133
Arithmetical skills after stroke, 41
Arm, paralysed, 51
  danger to, 51
Arteriogram, subtraction, 13
Aspirin, 15
  and blood clotting, 15, 16
Atherosclerosis, 12, 133
  causes, 15, 33
Bed rest, 47
  effects, 47
Bed, 47, 50
  rolling over in, 50
  sitting up in, 52
Blood, 11, 13

  coagulation, 13
  function, 11
  pressure checks, 17, 23, 33

Body image, 133
Brain, 11, 14, 18
Brain damage, 27, 29
  assessing degree of, 71, 73
  difference between the two
    sides, 39, 40, 41, 42
  extra-pyramidal system, 36
  functions of different parts, 35
  motor area, 35
  oxygen supply, 11
  pyramidal system, 36
  sensory area, 35, 37
  silent areas, 35
  visual area, 35
Brainstem, 134

CT scan, 134
Carbon monoxide, 15
Cardiovascular, 134
Carers, 102, 103
  guilt, 103
  overburdening, 102, 104
  privacy, 108
  rights, 102
  stress, 109, 110
  time off, 107
Carotid arteries, 12, 16, 31, 134